Update Gastroenterology 1996

John Libbey Eurotext
127, avenue de la République
92120 Montrouge
Tél. : 46 73 06 60

John Libbey and Company Ltd
13, Smiths Yard, Summerley Street
London SW18 4HR, England
Tel. : 1 947 27 77

John Libbey CIC
Via L. Spallanzani, 11
00161, Rome, Italie
Tel. : 06 862 289

© John Libbey Eurotext, 1996
ISBN : 2-7420-0150-6

Il est interdit de reproduire intégralement ou partiellement le présent ouvrage - loi du 11 mars 1957 - sans autorisation de l'éditeur ou du Centre Français du Copyright, 6 *bis*, rue Gabriel-Laumain, 75010 Paris, France.

Update Gastroenterology 1996

Edited by
J.P. Galmiche

Postgraduate Course 1996
Paris, November 3rd

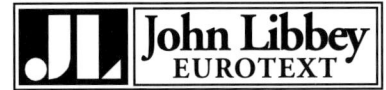

The publication of this book was made possible
thanks to the support from the Takeda Laboratories

Contents

Foreword
G.N.J. Tytgat IX

Presidential address
J.P. Galmiche XI

Evolving concepts in gastroenterology

Neuroimmune functions in the gastrointestinal tract
S.M. Collins, K. Jacobson 3

Intestinal infection
M.J.G. Farthing 13

Gene therapy: basic concepts and applications in gastrointestinal diseases
H.E. Blum, S. Wieland, F. von Weizsäcker 33

Vaccinating against *Helicobacter pylori* infections: reality and perspectives
A. Labigne, R. Ferrero 49

Recent advances in gastrointestinal oncology

Helicobacter pylori, gastric cancer and gastric lymphoma
S.G.M. Meuwissen, E.J. Kuipers 57

Octreoscan scintigraphy in endocrine gastroenteropancreatic tumors
G. Cadiot, R. Lebtahi, D. Le Guludec, M. Mignon 67

Progress in the treatment of liver metastases
T. Sauerbruch, R. Caspari, T. Heinicke, J. Metzger 79

Lynch syndrome (HNPCC): application to the prevention of colorectal cancer
H.J. Järvinen 89

Recent advances in gastrointestinal pharmacology and therapeutics

Modulation of visceral sensitivity
F. Azpiroz 99

Antidiarrheal therapy
G.J. Krejs 111

Prokinetic compounds
C. Scarpignato 115

Advances in medical therapy of inflammatory bowel disease
P. Rutgeerts, S. Vermeire 143

Recent advances in gastrointestinal surgery

Gastroesophageal reflux disease and esophageal motility disorders
L. Lundell 157

Adjuvant therapy and surgery of esophageal cancer
L. Bonavina, A. Peracchia 167

Repair of the anal sphincter
M.A. Kamm 175

List of contributors

Azpiroz F., Digestive System Research Unit, Hospital General Vall d'Hebron, Autonomous University of Barcelona, 08035 Barcelona, Spain.

Blum H.E., Department of Medicine II, University of Freiburg, Hugstetter Strasse 55, D.-79106 Freiburg, Germany.

Bonavina L., Department of General and Oncologic Surgery, University of Milan, Ospedale Maggiore Policlinico, IRCCS, Milano, Italy.

Cadiot G., Service d'Hépato-Gastroentérologie, CHU Bichat-Claude-Bernard, 16, rue Henri-Huchard, 75877 Paris Cedex 18, France.

Caspari R., Department of General Internal Medicine, Sigmund-Freud-Strasse 25, 53105 Bonn, Germany.

Collins S.M., Division of Gastroenterology, Department of Medicine, Intestinal Diseases Research Unit, McMaster University, Hamilton, Ontario, L8N 3Z5, Canada.

Farthing M.J.G., Digestive Diseases Research Centre, St Bartholomew's and the Royal London School of Medicine and Dentistry, Charterhouse Square, London EC1M 6QB, United Kingdom.

Ferrero R., Unité de Pathogénie Bactérienne des Muqueuses, INSERM U 389, Institut Pasteur, 25, rue du Docteur-Roux, 75724 Paris Cedex 15, France.

Heinicke T., Department of General Internal Medicine, Sigmund-Freud-Strasse 25, 53105 Bonn, Germany.

Jacobson K., Division of Gastroenterology, Department of Pediatrics, Intestinal Diseases Research Unit, McMaster University, Hamilton, Ontario, L8N 3Z5, Canada.

Järvinen H.J., Second Department of Surgery, University Central Hospital, Helsinki, Finland.

Kamm M.A., Physiology Unit, St Mark's Hospital, Northwick Park, Watford Road, Harrow, Middlesex HA1 3UJ, United Kingdom.

Krejs G.J., Department of Medicine, Karl-Franzens University, Graz, Austria.

Kuipers E.J., Department of Gastroenterology, University Hospital of the Vrije Universiteit, Amsterdam, The Netherlands.

Labigne A., Unité de Pathogénie Bactérienne des Muqueuses, INSERM U 389, Institut Pasteur, 25, rue du Docteur-Roux, 75724 Paris Cedex 15, France.

Lebtahi R., Service de Médecine Nucléaire, CHU Bichat-Claude-Bernard, 16, rue Henri-Huchard, 75877 Paris Cedex 18, France.

Le Guludec D., Service de Médecine Nucléaire, CHU Bichat-Claude-Bernard, 16, rue Henri-Huchard, 75877 Paris Cedex 18, France.

Lundell L., Department of Surgery, Sahlgren's University Hospital, University of Gothenburg, S-41345 Gothenburg, Sweden.

Metzger J., Department of General Internal Medicine, Sigmund-Freud-Strasse 25, 53105 Bonn, Germany.

Meuwissen S.G.M., Department of Gastroenterology, University Hospital of the Vrije Universiteit, Amsterdam, The Netherlands.

Mignon M., Service d'Hépato-Gastroentérologie, CHU Bichat-Claude-Bernard, 16, rue Henri-Huchard, 75877 Paris Cedex 18, France.

Peracchia A., Department of General and Oncologic Surgery, University of Milan, Ospedale Maggiore Policlinico, IRCCS, Milano, Italy.

Rutgeerts P., Department of Medicine, University Hospital, 3000 Leuven, Belgium.

Sauerbruch T., Department of General Internal Medicine, Sigmund-Freud-Strasse 25, 53105 Bonn, Germany.

Scarpignato C., Institute of Pharmacology, School of Medicine and Dentistry, Maggiore University Hospital, 43100 Parma, Italy.

Vermeire S., Department of Medicine, University Hospital, 3000 Leuven, Belgium.

von Weizsäcker F., Department of Medicine II, University of Freiburg, Hugstetter Strasse 55, D-79106 Freiburg, Germany.

Wieland S., Department of Medicine II, University of Freiburg, Hugstetter Strasse 55, D-79106 Freiburg, Germany.

Foreword

The European Association for Gastroenterology and Endoscopy, EAGE, had a long tradition of organizing annual scientific meetings with an especially heavy emphasis on clinically related gastroenterological, hepatological and endoscopic diseases as well as related problems. The restructuring of European educational activities occurred a few years ago due to the creation of the United European Federation. At that time, the emphasis of the EAGE switched to the organisation of top level postgraduate courses during the annual European meeting. Additionally, several smaller scale regional gastrointestinal-related meetings were organized by or carried out under the auspices of the EAGE. Focusing on the annual postgraduate course corresponds well with the aims of the EAGE which are to foster basic and clinical research in gastroenterology-hepatology-endoscopy. The Governing Board of the EAGE, composed of top clinicians and researchers in gastroenterology in Europe, is ultimately responsible for the selection of topics and speakers for the annual postgraduate course. The Board's standing and expertise guarantees a high level of clinical and basic teaching.

In the past, a syllabus was produced which was distributed at the time of the postgraduate course. For the first time this year, through the initiatives of Pr Galmiche, EAGE chairman and chief responsible for the Postgraduate Course 1996, the course proceedings are published in full. This will enable us to maintain a permanent record of state-of-the-art lecturing on the various selected topics. The content of *Update Gastroenterology 1996* is a superb testimony of the cutting edge developments in gastroenterology. The very latest information is given on neuroimmune function, infections, gene therapy, *H. pylori* vaccination, *H. pylori* related cancer/lymphoma, endocrine tumor detection, liver metastasis, Lynch syndromes, visceral sensitivity, antidiarrheal and prokinetic drugs, inflammatory bowel disease, reflux disease, esophageal cancer, sphincter dysfunction and repair. Indeed an impressive collection of topics, discussed by the most qualified clinical investigators in Europe.

We hope that this important step will be the beginning of a long series of EAGE Postgraduate Course proceedings, that they will grow to become a personal library for each gastroenterologist at easy hand reach to check and consult the current state of knowledge in the various gastrointestinal related areas. Creating a permanent printed report of the postgraduate course will contribute substantially to enhancing further its high levels of teaching and impact on the European gastrointestinal community. May this very first, but important step be the beginning of a long lasting tradition illustrating the ultimate goal of the EAGE which is continuous state of the art education.

On behalf of the EAGE Governing Board,

G.N.J. Tytgat

Presidential address

Being elected President of the European Association for Gastroenterology and Endoscopy (EAGE) is an unquestionable honour, but the responsibility behind it is certainly greater. In the recent years, indeed, our Society, the EAGE, has played a key role in the development of European Gastroenterology. Its Past-Presidents have all been bright clinicians and established scientists who adopted a far-seeing policy thus allowing the Society to become an enthusiastic and stimulating forum of scientific and personal exchanges. There is however a long way to run for European Gastroenterology to reach the high standard which is both desirable for a scientific discipline and needed to counterbalance American Gastroenterology. Indeed, although the scientific level of several European teams is rather excellent, it must be recognised that data are disseminated mainly through « non European » means, *i.e.* national Societies and journals or North American Meetings and publications. Our aim should therefore be the promotion of European Gastroenterology *via* Europe. In this connection, we should continue the efforts, already undertaken during the last few years, to increase the scientific level and the originality of the papers presented at the United European Gastroenterology Week (UEGW) and to enhance the spread and the impact factor of the leading European journals.

What can in practical terms a President of EAGE do? First of all, he can emphasise his firm belief on a European Society whose individual members are capable of exceeding National frontiers. The power of our Society will depend on the number of the affiliated members. Although our number is already considerable, it is crucial that the opinion leaders of each Country belong to the Society and make efforts to urge European clinicians and scientists to join us. Only then can our number reach the critical mass necessary to represent European Gastroenterology all over the World. I consider this objective amongst my priorities and would like my Presidency be judged also on the basis of the results achieved in this field.

An additional important aim of EAGE is to develop gastrointestinal education in Europe. To this end, starting from 1992, several Post-graduate Courses have been organised during the UEGW, including the last one held in Berlin the past September. There, more than 800 attendants made it a great success and clearly showed that there is both a need and an appreciation of such educational events. In addition, we would like to organise, as we did in the past, Post-graduate Courses outside the UEGW in different European Countries, including the East ones. This is obviously a « scientific » way to unify the « two Europes » within only one European Society. Besides the present one, several Courses under the auspices of the EAGE are scheduled for the next year. These courses, specifically devoted to young scientists and clinicians, will surely encourage friendship and cooperation among the members of different European teams.

In summary, a lot of work is still to be done. However, the enthusiasm of the members of the EAGE Governing Board and the successful trends of the Society represent for me the more exciting stimulus. We will all be successful provided our number grows. Therefore, please, join us and win!

Jean Paul Galmiche
President of EAGE
and Director of the Post-graduate Course

Evolving concepts
in gastroenterology

Neuroimmune functions in the gastrointestinal tract

S.M. Collins[1], K. Jacobson[2]

Division of Gastroenterology, Departments of Medicine[1] and Pediatrics[2], Intestinal Diseases Research Unit, McMaster University, Hamilton, Ontario, L8N 3Z5, Canada

Summary

Structural studies have shown close approximation of nerves and various immune cell types in the gut. These cells possess biologically active receptors for a variety of neurotransmitters which can thereby alter immune function. Conversely, nerves or their support cells such as glia, possess receptors for a variety of ligands produced by immune or inflammatory cells and include cytokines, lymphokines, prostaglandins and leukotrienes. These observations provide the structural basis upon which to consider bi-directional interactions between nerves and immune cells. In addition, the scope of neuroimmune interactions can be broadened to include the brain, which through the neuroendocrine pathways of the brain-gut axis can either be influenced by immune activation in the gut, or modulate immune or inflammatory processes in the gut. This review will address bi-directional interactions between nerves and immune cells in clinical contexts of food allergy, intestinal pseudo-obstruction and inflammatory bowel disease.

Overview

The structural basis for neuroimmune interactions

Over the past twenty years there has been a growing body of evidence demonstrating the presence of receptors for neuropeptides on immunocompetent cells (for review, see [1]). The innervation of lymphoid tissue [2] and the close approximation of nerves and lamina propria cells such as mast cells [3] illustrate the feasibility of neural modulation of immune function in the gut.

The interaction between immune cells and nerves is bi-directional. Studies in the brain have shown the presence of, for example, cytokines on nerves [4] using direct ligand binding studies. In the gut, the presence of cytokine receptors on enteric nerves has been invoked on the basis of functional studies using crude synaptosomes prepared from the intestinal myenteric plexus of rat. In these studies, cytokines IL-1β and TNF-α suppressed the release of noradrenaline from synaptosomes prepared from myenteric plexus; the action of IL-1β and part of the action of TNF-α were inhibited by the IL-1 receptor antagonist, suggesting the presence of the IL-1 receptor on adrenergic nerves in the gut (for review, see [5]).

The scope of neuroimmune interactions as they relate to the gut

Neuroimmune interactions are not restricted to cells within the gut, but also occur in extrinsic nerves, such as the superior cervical ganglion. Freidin *et al.* have shown that exposure of cultured explants from rat superior cervical ganglion increased the content of the neuropeptide substance P by an action mediated *via* Schwann cells, whereas another cytokine Leukemia Inhibitory Factor (LIF) exerted its effects directly on ganglion cells and on pure neuronal cultures [6].

The scope of neuro-immune actions pertaining to gut function have been extended to the brain. Fargeas *et al.* [7] showed that IL-1β administered to the brain stimulated colonic motility in dogs; the action could not be mimicked by administering larger doses of the cytokine peripherally and were blocked by the IL-1 receptor antagonist given centrally. Similarly, McHugh *et al.* showed that the anorexia that occurs following experimental colitis is mediated in part by IL-1 in the central nervous system, as well as by IL-1 in the periphery [8]. Thus, cytokines released from sources such as astroglia interact the central neurons to modulate feeding behaviour or gut physiology. Studies addressing the ability of stress to modify inflammatory process in the gut [9] provide additional evidence that the scope of neuroimmune interactions extends well beyond the gut to alter intestinal function.

The clinical contexts of neuro-immune interactions

Type I immediate hypersensitivity reactions
Food allergy

Diarrhea and abdominal cramping may accompany food allergy. Radiological studies in man have shown that exposure to an allergenic food in patients with food allergy results in a rapid acceleration of the gastroduodenal transit of barium. Malatesta *et al.* showed that mouth to caecum transit time is accelerated after oral food antigen in patients with irritable bowel syndrome-like symptoms and positive skin tests for food allergens when compared to a skin prick negative IBS group. The transit time was attenuated by pretreatment with oral cromoglycate, implicating mast cells as the mediator of these changes. Similar observations have been made in rats sensitized to ovalbumin [10]. Presentation of antigen at one site in the gut caused extensive changes in motility that were apparent at sites that had not been exposed to the antigen. Since motor function over large segments requires an intact enteric circuitry, the widespread response to localized application of food antigen implicates interactions between mast cells and nerves. This has been shown electrophysiologically *in vivo* in animals sensitized by previous infection with the nematode *Trichinella spiralis* [11]. In addition, in ovalbumin-sensitized rats it has also been shown that antigen stimulation in the sensitized bowel activates afferent nerves [12] and involves substance P and 5-hydroxytryptamine (5-HT) and vagal afferents [13]. In addition, pretreatment of sensitized rats with the IL-1 receptor antagonist by intraperitoneal injection abrogated the motor response to antigen exposure [14]. *In vitro* studies have shown that the stimulation of mast cells by anti-IgE antibody causes persistent firing of neurons in the gut. Thus, neuroimmune interactions may constitute part of the process that follows the ingestion of food allergen in sensitized patients with food allergy.

Autoimmune interactions
Intestinal pseudo-obstruction or achalasia

Intestinal pseudo-obstruction is a clinical term that encompasses a broad range of pathogenetic processes that include a visceral myopathy, a familial degenerative syndrome as well as a neuropathic variety. In latter, there is a subgroup of patients who develop the syndrome as part of a paraneoplastic syndrome [15]. Based on recent findings it is likely that this occurs as a result of an autoimmune reaction directed against enteric nerves, and as such shares a common basis with connective tissue disorders such as scleroderma, or achalasia syndromes. This is based on the discovery of anti-neuronal antibodies in this subgroup of patients with pseudo-obstruction and the subsequent demonstration that these antibodies can alter neural function. Caras *et al.* [16] recently investigated the effects of IgG containing anti-neuronal antibody (ANAb) on neural components of the ascending excitatory reflex (AER) contraction and peristalsis in the isolated guinea pig ileum. The ANAb inhibited the AER by about 60 % and occasionally reduced the frequency of peristalsis by about 50 % but had little effect on amplitude. Immunofluorescence showed uptake of gANAb, but not control IgG, initially in the deep muscular plexus after 15 minutes and subsequently into some myenteric neurons, thereby altering neurotransmission in a manner similar to that observed following the addition of hexamethonium to the preparation.

Inflammatory bowel diseases

It has long been recognized that in human inflammatory bowel disease (IBD), inflammation causes structural changes in enteric neural axons and ganglia [17-19]. Changes in neurotransmitter content has provided discrepant data with increases reported in a variety of peptides including a decrease in VIP and an increase in substance P in IBD [20] whereas others have reported an increase in VIP [21]. Autonomic balance is altered in IBD and does not appear to change after colectomy for colitis suggesting it may be a primary rather than secondary phenomenon [22]. The sympathetic neurotransmitter content is also altered [23, 24] in colitis. Rectal sensitivity to distension is increased, thus providing functional data suggestive of neural involvement. In these examples, nerves are involved by the inflammatory process as « innocent by-standers » and likely influenced by inflammatory cell products or immune activation [25]. Intestinal inflammation due to Crohn's disease is associated with malnutrition and growth retardation in children; part of this reflects a decrease in food intake. This taken together with the observation that there are structural abnormalities in the CNS reported in IBD [26] raise the possibility that intestinal inflammation alters brain function to reduce appetite.

The effects of inflammation on nerves

The above-described observations are also supported by work in animal studies where neurotransmitter release from myenteric nerves is impaired in the presence of inflammation. There is a marked suppression of both norepinephrine and acetylcholine from myenteric nerves [27, 28] in the inflamed intestine of *T. spiralis* rats. Also in TNB induced colitis we have also found that inflammation reduces the release from the myenteric plexus but not only in the inflamed distal colon but also in the non-inflamed transverse colon and ileum [29]. These actions are mediated at least in part by IL-1β and perhaps by leukemia inhibitory factor [30]. Several cytokines have been shown to exert influence on myenteric nerve function. Some studies have raised the possibility that there is a source of endogenous IL-1 within the myenteric plexus as the actions of LPS [31] and of exogenous IL-1β are mediated by endogenous IL-1 [32]. Putative cellular sources of IL-1 in the plexus include macrophage-like cells [33], resident macrophages and enteroglia [34]. The latter have been isolated and cultured from the rat GI tract and have been shown to release cytokines such as IL-6 on exposure to IL-1β. We hypothesized that enteroglia EGC, strategically located within the ENS, are themselves subject to the influence of neurotransmitter, thus creating a bi-directional neuro-immune axis. We studied the effects of adrenergic and cholinergic neurotransmitter, and of substance P on interleukin-6 (IL-6) expression in EGC clones *in vitro*. EGC clones were raised from single cells isolated from the small intestine of healthy adult rats. The purity of the clones was morphologically and immunocytochemically confirmed, using antibodies directed against GFAP and S-100. The clones were stimulated with adrenergic and muscarinic agonists as well as substance P for 24 hours, and IL-6 bioactivity was determined from cell-free tissue-culture supernatants using the B9 cell proliferation assay. We were able to show that adrenergic agonists induce IL-6 synthesis in EGC whereas muscarinic agonists and substance P were without effect. Based on these findings, we propose that EGC act as intermediates between the enteric immune and nervous system, and thus play a pivotal role in the bi-directional neuro-immune axis in the enteric nervous system.

We have extended our work to include the brain. Rats with acute TNB-induced colitis exhibit a reduction in food intake and body weight [35] that cannot be attributed to general malaise [36]. It is mediated in part *via* a delay in gastric emptying [37] and involves both central (CNS) and peripheral interleukin-1 receptors [8]. These studies provide an example of neuro-immune interactions occurring in the context of inflammation and involving the central nervous system as an « innocent by-stander ». Studies involving stress show that the CNS may also be involved as an active participant to modulate intestinal inflammation (see below).

The effect of nerves on inflammation

There are several lines of observation that suggest a more active or participatory role of nerves in the inflammatory process in IBD. For example, historically, denervation of the pelvic colon was used to treat refractory colitis before the availability of potent antiinflammatory drugs [38]. The apparent therapeutic benefit afforded by clonidine [39], nicotine [40] and lidocaine [41], taken together with the documentation of autonomic imbalance in IBD patients that persists after colectomy [22, 42], raise the possibility that nerve may modulate intestinal inflammation. In addition, the possible relationship between stress and relapses of IBD raises the possibility that neuromodulation of intestinal inflammation may involve the central nervous system. These possibilities have been addressed in animal models of intestinal inflammation.

Patients with IBD may report that their condition first presented at a time of emotional stress while others may report that established disease may relapse at times of stress. Two recent reports using animal models support these claims. First, Gue *et al.* showed that rats subjected to stress immediately prior the induction of colitis using TNB experienced an enhanced acute inflammatory response, as reflected by myeloperoxidase activity or histological damage [43]. In a previous study, McHugh *et al.* showed that stress reactivated the inflammatory process in rats whose colitis, induced six weeks previously, was in full histological remission [44]. Although the stress-induced reactivation did not produce a full blown colitis, the study illustrated the ability of stress to rekindle the dormant inflammatory process. The basis for the rekindling of the inflammatory process by stress could reflect a number of mechanisms. Stress may favor bacterial translocation across the gut facilitated by stress-induced increases in permeability [45] and a reduction in mucin production [46]. It is also possible that the rekindling of the inflammatory process reflects a direct neuro-immune interaction. For example, stress was accompanied by a reduction in the expression of mRNA for IL-1β which was elevated six weeks post TNB colitis. Although IL-1 is generally recognized as a pro-inflammatory cytokine, it is also known to display anti-inflammatory actions during later stages of inflammation. Thus, the inflammatory process could have been reactivated by de-repressing the protective effect of IL-1. This interpretation is speculative and needs to be tested directly in the model under study. Thus, further work is required to fully understand the mechanism underlying stress-induced enhancement or reactivation of intestinal inflammation, as it may yield a new therapeutic approach.

Substance P has long been implicated as a pro-inflammatory peptide [47]. Its receptor is upregulated in lymphoid tissue and on blood vessels in Crohn's disease [48] - both strategically important sites considering the inflammatory actions of the peptide. In animal models, the role of substance P in intestinal inflammation has been elucidated. In small intestinal inflammation induced by nematode infection, there is an 8-fold increase in immunoreactive substance P [49]. The increase in substance P is evident at the transcriptional level since it was accompanied by an increase in the Preprotachykinin gene that encodes substance P [50]. If tissue from the inflamed segment is treated with the neurotoxin, scorpion venom, the substance P is depleted, indicating that the increase in substance P content is of neural origin [49]. Treatment of rats with capsaicin prior to infection prevented the increase in substance P indicating that it is present primarily in primary afferents [49]. An increase in immunoreactive substance P could be induced in the tissue following exposure to IL-1β [51] and since treatment of infected rats with an IL-1 receptor antagonist abrogated the increase in substance P, we concluded that this cytokine mediates the change in substance P levels in the inflamed gut [52].

In addition to the increase in substance P, its bioavailability in the inflamed gut is substantially increased as neutral endopeptidase, its main degrading enzyme, is substantially down-regulated during inflammation [53]. Thus, the gut is primed to receive the full biological impact of any released substance P. Considering its pro-inflammatory properties, any release of this peptide in the gut is likely to enhance the inflammatory response.

To evaluate that possibility, nematode-infected mice were treated with anti-substance P antibody or antagonist during the course of infection and this significantly attenuated the inflammation [54], implicating substance P as a mediator of inflammation in this model. Based on this result, one might expect to see that capsaicin depletion of substance P containing nerves would also ameliorate inflammation but the several groups have shown that the converse is true. That is, that chronic capsaicin treatment to deplete primary afferent nerves of substance P significantly worsened the inflammation seen in nematode-infected rats [49] as well as in TNB-induced colitis [55]. These results indicate that although locally released substance P is pro-inflammatory when released antidromically from sensory nerves, and clearly contributes to the inflammatory process in models studied to date, the neural afferent neural circuit is protective and anti-inflammatory as shown by the capsaicin data. The protective sensory neurotransmitter is likely calcitonin gene related peptide, CGRP, as administration of exogenous peptide improved inflammation in animal model of inflammation [56].

In terms of the autonomic nervous system, our preliminary studies in animals suggest that sympathetic nerves are protective against inflammation as chemical sympathectomy results in a deterioration in inflammation due to TNB colitis (unpublished). This is consistent with the report that the adrenergic agonist clonidine improves colitis in man [39].

We had suspected that the integrity of intrinsic nerves might be important in modulating inflammation or at least rendering the gut more susceptible to inflammation. The reason for this hypothesis is based on the fact that Crohn's disease frequently recurs at the anastomotic site following resection. We were unable to demonstrate a greater degree of inflammation at either side of the anastomotic line in animals with experimental colitis (unpublished observation). In other studies where we had excluded a segment of gut by creating a Thiery-Vella loop, we found that inflammation induced by TNB or acetic acid was greater in that segment compared to the gut in-continuity. This may be due to disruption of the intrinsic nerves or to differences in the bacterial content of the gut lumen.

References

1. Payan DG, McGillis JP, Goetzl EJ. Neuroimmunology. *Adv Immunol* 1986; 39: 299-323.
2. Felten DL, Felten SY, Carlson SL, Olschowka JA, Livnat S. Noradrenergic and peptidergic innervation of lymphoid. *J Immunol* 1985; 135: 755s-65s.
3. Stead RH, Tomioka M, Quinonez G, Simon GT, Felten SY, Bienenstock J. Intestinal mucosal mast cells in normal and nematode infected rat intestines are in intimate contact with peptidergic nerves. *Proc Natl Acad Sci USA* 1987; 84: 2975-9.
4. Takao T, Tracey DE, Mitchell WM, DeSouza EB. Interleukin-1 receptors in mouse brain: characterization and neuronal localization. *Endocrinology* 1990; 127: 3070-7.
5. Collins SM, Hurst SM, Main C, Stanley E, Khan I, Blennerhassett P, Swain M. Effect of inflammation of enteric nerves. Cytokine-induced changes in neurotransmitter content and release. *Ann N Y Acad Sci* 1992; 664: 415-24.
6. Freidin M, Kessler JA. Cytokine regulation of substance P expression in sympathetic neurons. *Proc Natl Acad Sci USA* 1991; 88: 3200-3.

7. Fargeas MJ, Fioramonti J, Bueno L. Central action of interleukin 1 beta on intestinal motility in rats: mediation by two mechanisms. *Gastroenterology* 1993; 104: 377-83.
8. McHugh KJ, Collins SM, Weingarten HP. Central interleukin-1 receptors contribute to suppression of feeding after acute colitis in the rat. *Am J Physiol* 1994; 266: R1659-63.
9. Ito Y. The absence of resistance in congenitally athymic nude mice toward infection with the intestinal nematode, *Trichuris muris*: resistance restored by lymphoid cell transfer. *Int J Parasitol* 1991; 21: 65-9.
10. Scott RB, Diamant SC, Gall GA. Motility effects of intestinal anaphylaxis in the rat. *Am J Physiol* 1988; 255: G505-11.
11. Palmer JM, Castro GA. Anamnestic stimulus-specific myoelectrical responses associated with intestinal immunity in the rat. *Am J Physiol* 1986; 250: G266-73.
12. Fargeas MJ, Fioramonti J, Bueno L. Involvement of capsaicin-sensitive afferent nerves in the intestinal motor alterations induced by intestinal anaphylaxis in rats. *Int Arch Allergy Immunol* 1993; 101: 190-5.
13. Castex N, Fioramonti J, Fargeas MJ, More J, Bueno L. Role of 5-HT3 receptors and afferent fibers in the effects of mast cell degranulation on colonic motility in rats. *Gastroenterology* 1994; 107: 976-84.
14. Theodorou V, Fioramonti J, Bueno L. Recombinant interleukin-1 receptor antagonist protein prevents sensitization and intestinal anaphylaxis in guinea pigs. *Life Sci* 1993; 53: 733-8.
15. Krishnamurthy S, Schufffler MD, Belic L, Schweid AI. An inflammatory axonopathy of the myenteric plexus producing a rapidly progressive intestinal pseudoobstruction. *Gastroenterology* 1986; 90: 754-8.
16. Caras SD, McCallum RW, Brashear SR, Smith TK. The effect of human anti-neuronal antibodies on the ascending excitatory reflex and peristalsis in the guinea pig ileum. *Gastroenterology* 1996; in press.
17. Dvorak AM, Connell AB, Dickersin GR. Crohn's disease, a scanning electron microscopic study. *Hum Pathol* 1979; 10: 165-77.
18. Dvorak AM, Osage JE, Monahan RA, Dickersin GR. Crohn's disease: transmission electron microscopic studies. III Target tissues. Proliferation of and injury to smooth muscle and the autonomic nervous system. *Hum Pathol* 1980; 11: 620-34.
19. Davis DR, Dockerty MB, Mayo CB. The myenteric plexus in regional enteritis: a study of the number of ganglion cells in the ileum in 24 cases. *Surg Gynecol Obstet* 1953; 101: 208-16.
20. Koch TR, Carney A, Go VLW. Distribution and quantification of gut neuropeptides in normal intestine and inflammatory bowel diseases. *Dig Dis Sci* 1987; 32: 369-76.
21. O'Morain C, Bishop AE, McGregor GP, Levi AJ, Bloom SR, Polak JM, Peters TJ. Vasoactive intestinal peptide concentrations and immunocytochemical studies in rectal biopsies from patients with inflammatory bowel disease. *Gut* 1984; 25: 56-61.
22. Lindgren S, Stewenius J, Sjolund K, Lilja B, Sundkvist G. Autonomic vagal nerve dysfunction in patients with ulcerative colitis. *Scand J Gastroenterol* 1993; 28: 638-42.
23. Kyosola K, Penttila O, Salaspuro M. Rectal mucosal adrenergic innervation and enterochromaffin cells in ulcerative colitis and irritable colon. *Scand J Gastroenterol* 1977; 12: 363-67.
24. Penttila O, Kyosola K, Klinge E, Ahonen A, Tallqvist G. Studies on rectal mucosal catecholamines in ulcerative colitis. *Ann Clin Res* 1975; 7: 32-6.
25. Geboes K, Rutgeerts P, Ectors N, Mebis J, Penninckx F, Vantrappen G, Desmet VJ. Major histocompatibility class II expression on the small intestinal nervous system in Crohn's disease. *Gastroenterology* 1992; 103: 439-47.
26. Andus T, Geissler A, Roth M, Kullmann F, Caesar P, Held P, Gross S, Feuerbah S, Scholmerich J. Small focal white matter lesions in the brain of patients with inflammatory bowel disease - another extraintestinal manifestation? *Gastroenterology* 1994; 106: A645 (Abstract).

27. Collins SM, Blennerhassett PA, Blennerhassett MG, Vermillion DL. Impaired acetylcholine release from the myenteric plexus of Trichinella-infected rats. *Am J Physiol* 1989; 257: G898-903.
28. Swain MG, Blennerhassett PA, Collins SM. Impaired sympathetic nerve function in the inflamed rat intestine. *Gastroenterology* 1991; 100: 675-82.
29. Jacobson K, McHugh K, Collins SM. Experimental colitis alters myenteric nerve function at inflamed and noninflamed sites in the rat. *Gastroenterology* 1995; 109: 718-22.
30. Van Assche G, Collins SM. Leukemia inhibitory factor is a mediator of the action of interleukin-1β in rat myenteric of rat myenteric plexus. *Gastroenterology* 1996; in press.
31. Stanley E, Stead R, Collins SM. *E. coli* endotoxin exerts a biphasic effect on acetylcholine release from rat myenteric plexus. *Gastroenterology* 1992; 102: 4: A700 (Abstract).
32. Main C, Blennerhassett P, Collins SM. Human recombinant interleukin 1 beta suppresses acetylcholine release from rat myenteric plexus. *Gastroenterology* 1993; 104: 1648-54.
33. Ruhl A, Berezin I, Collins SM. Involvement of eicosanoids and macrophage-like cells in cytokine-mediated changes in rat myenteric nerves. *Gastroenterology* 1995; 109: 1852-62.
34. Ruhl A, Collins SM. Enteroglial cells are an integral part of the neuroimmune axis in the gut. *Gastroenterology* 1995.
35. McHugh K, Castonguay TW, Collins SM, Weingarten HP. Characterization of suppression of food intake following acute colon inflammation in the rat. *Am J Physiol* 1993; 265: R1001-5.
36. McHugh KJ, Weingarten HP, Keenan C, Wallace J, Collins SM. On the suppression of food intake in experimental colitis in the rat. *Am J Physiol* 1993; 264: R871-6.
37. McHugh K, Weingarten HP, Collins SM. The role of delayed gastric emptying in anorexia induced by intestinal inflammation in the rat. *Soc Neurosci* 1991; 17 (1): 493 (Abstract).
38. Shafiroff GP, Hinton J. Denervation of the pelvic colon for ulcerative colitis. *Surg Forum* 1950; 134-9.
39. Lechin F, van der Dijs B, Insausti CL. Treatment of ulcerative colitis with clonidine. *J Clin Pharmacol* 1985; 25: 255-62.
40. Koide M, Kawahara Y, Tsuda T, Nakayama I, Yokoyama M. Expression of nitric oxide synthase by cytokines in vascular smooth muscle cells. *Hypertension* 1994; 23: 145-8.
41. Bjorck S, Dahlstrom A, Johansson L, Ahlman H. Treatment of the mucosa with local anaesthetics in ulcerative colitis. *Agents Actions* 1992; 10: C61-72.
42. Lindgren S, Lilja B, Rosén I, Sundkvist G. Disturbed autonomic nerve function in patients with Crohn's disease. *Scand J Gastroenterol* 1991; 26: 361-6.
43. Gue M, Fioramonti J, Bonhomme C, Del Rio C, Junien J, Bueno L. Chronic partial restraint stress enhances trinitrobenzene sufonic acid-induced colitis in rats. *Gastroenterology* 1995; 108: A553 (Abstract).
44. McHugh K, Weingarten HP, Khan I, Riddell R, Collins SM. Stress-induced exacerbation of experimental colitis in the rat. *Gastroenterology* 1993; 104 (4): A1051 (Abstract).
45. Saunders PR, Kosecka U, McKay DM, Bienenstock JB, Perdue MH. Stress increases intestinal epithelial permeability, stimulates ion secretion, and alters enteric nerve function in the rat. *Gastroenterology* 1993; 104: A1061 (Abstract).
46. Rubio CA, Huang CB. Quantification of the sulphomucin-producing cell population of the colonic mucosa during protracted stress in rats. *In vivo* 1992; 6: 81-4.
47. Payan DG. Neuropeptides and inflammation: the role of substance P. *Annu Rev Med* 1989; 40: 341-52.
48. Mantyh CR, Gates TS, Zimmerman RP, Welton ML, Passaro EP, Jr, Vigna SR, Maggio JE, Kruger L, Mantyh PW. Receptor binding sites for substance P, but not substance K or neuromedin K, are expressed in high concentrations by arterioles, venules, and lymph nodules in surgical specimens obtained from patients with ulcerative colitis and Crohn's disease. *Proc Natl Acad Sci USA* 1988; 85: 3235-9.

49. Swain MG, Agro A, Blennerhassett P, Stanisz A, Collins SM. Increased levels of substance P in the myenteric plexus of Trichinella-infected rats. *Gastroenterology* 1992; 102: 1913-9.
50. Khan I, Collins SM. Expression of substance P mRNA in the inflamed intestine of rat. *Gastroenterology* 1993; 104 (4): A833 (Abstract).
51. Hurst SM, Stanisz AM, Sharkey KA, Collins SM. Interleukin 1 beta-induced increase in substance P in rat myenteric plexus. *Gastroenterology* 1993; 105: 1754-60.
52. Collins SM, Blennerhassett P, Hurst S, Khan I, Thompson RC. The role of endogenous interleukin-1B in enteric nerve and muscle changes in the inflamed nematode-infected rat intestine. *Gastroenterology* 1992; 102: 4: A608 (Abstract).
53. Hwang L, Okamoto A, Leichter R, Collins SM, Bunnett NW. Neutral endopeptidase (NEP, EC 3. 4. 24. 11) is down regulated in the intestine by infection with Trichinella spiralis. *Gastroenterology* 1992; 102: 4: A927 (Abstract).
54. Agro A, Stanisz AM. Inhibition of murine intestinal inflammation by anti-substance P antibody. *Rev Immunol* 1993; 5: 120-6.
55. Reinshagen. Effect of capsaicin in TNB colitis. *Gastroenterology* 1996; in press.
56. Eysselein VE, Reinshagen M, Patel A, Davis W, Nast C, Sternini C. Calcitonin gene related peptide in inflammatory bowel disease and experimentally induced colitis. *Ann NY Acad Sci* 1992; 657: 319-27.

Intestinal infection

M.J.G. Farthing

Digestive Diseases Research Centre, St Bartholomew's and The Royal London School of Medicine and Dentistry, and Charterhouse Square, London EC1M 6BQ, UK

Summary

Infections of the gastrointestinal tract are the most common intestinal disorders. Although gut infections have their major impact in the developing world, the numbers of reported infections continue to increase in many industrialised countries including the United Kingdom and North America. This relates in part to the transmission of intestinal infection in food and underscores the continuing need to be vigilant in food production and food handling. In recent years, our knowledge on many aspects of intestinal infection has increased. New developments have occurred in our understanding of the epidemiology of these infections, new organisms have been discovered and new mechanisms of diarrhoea elucidated. The techniques of molecular genetics have permitted the development of new diagnostic approaches and through our appreciation of the pathogenesis and pathophysiology of infective diarrhoea, new treatments have emerged. Finally, the sophistication and efficacy of vaccines for enteric infection continue to improve, such that these should be available for the majority of important gut infections by the end of this millennium.

New epidemiology

Travellers

Infections of the gastrointestinal tract are most commonly acquired through ingestion of contaminated food and water, but may be transmitted by person to person contact. Travellers from the industrialised world to developing countries are at greatest risk and this includes military personnel as well as civilians [1-4]. Analysis of enteric pathogens in 432 military personnel in Saudi Arabia during operation Desert Shield identified an enteric pathogen in 49.5 % of troops with gastroenteritis [5]. Enterotoxigenic *Escherichia coli* (ETEC) was the most commonly isolated organism closely followed by *Shigella sonnei*.

A large number of these infections were resistant to standard antibiotics such as co-trimoxazole, tetracycline and amoxycillin, presumably related to the widespread use of these antibiotics in this geographic location. All bacterial isolates, however, were sensitive to the new quinolone antibiotics, norfloxacin and ciprofloxacin.

Food and drink

Food continues to be an important reservoir for intestinal infections and despite the political upheavals that followed the publicity about the high prevalence of *Salmonella enteritidis* phage type 4 in chickens and eggs, the number of reported salmonella infections continues to increase in the United Kingdom and little seems to have been done to control *Salmonella* sp. and *Campylobacter* sp. in chicken flocks [6, 7]. Heating food does not necessarily render it safe, since a variety of enteropathogens can survive in food at 50°C, which is too hot to touch [8]. Most enteropathogens survive well at refrigerator temperature (4°C) and for 24 hours in ice, even when placed in strong alcoholic drinks such as scotch whiskey and tequila [9]. Enteric pathogens such as salmonella, shigella and ETEC proliferate in milk but are inhibited in carbonated beverages and are rapidly killed in wine.

Swimming pools, seawater and freshwater lakes

Swimming has now become a dangerous recreational activity with respect to the acquisition of intestinal infections. Swimming pools are occasionally responsible for transmission, particularly of *Cryptosporidium parvum* and *Giardia lamblia* [10, 11]. Swimming pool water can become contaminated by the faeces of young children and the cysts of these parasites are able to survive even in chlorinated water for extended periods. Seawater may also be a danger to swimmers [12, 13]. Many beaches around the world are now contaminated with sewage and faecal micro-organisms. A recent survey of Ramsgate beach in Kent confirmed that diarrhoea and other abdominal symptoms were more common in bathers than non-bathers and that the coliform count failed to achieve European Community standards on 12 % of the sampling occasions [13]. Inland lakes and rivers are generally not approved for recreational swimming and are not routinely monitored. Recent evidence confirms that more than 80 % of fresh water locations that had been tested in Britain were contaminated with cyanobacterial toxins, for which the increasing use for nitrate and phosphate fertilisers and a series of long, hot summers are thought account [12, 14]. Holiday makers are advised to refer to the Heinz Good Beach Guide for up to date information on seawater contamination.

An outbreak of dysentery was recently described in swimmers using a freshwater lake in the state of Oregon, in the United States [15]. Two organisms were responsible, *Shigella sonnei* and *Enterohaemorrhagic E.coli*, serotype 0157: H7. Swimmers developed a self-limiting haemorrhagic colitis, a major risk factor being the swallowing of lakewater. It must be assumed that either the freshwater lake was contaminated with sewage or that the organisms had been released directly from a human reservoir.

Algal blooms

Algal blooms now constitute an important health risk world-wide [16]. Toxic phytoplankton blooms are associated with paralytic, diarrhoeal and amnesic shellfish poisoning and with histamine (scromboid), pufferfish and ciguatera fish poisoning. Algal blooms (red, green, golden, brown, bioluminescent) are widely distributed in marine, estuarine and inland waters in the Americas, Japan, South-East Asia and Australia. Increase in algal blooms has been attributed to a variety of environmental factors including a rise in sea temperatures, pollution and over-harvesting of fish and shellfish. The seasonality of cholera has been related to coastal algal blooms but the reservoir of cholera vibrios remained undetected until recently. However, a viable non-culturable form of *V. cholerae* has been found associated with certain varieties of surface marine life [17]. Under the conditions which favour algal blooms, *V. cholerae* reverts to its culturable and infectious state.

V. cholerae non-01 and the 8th cholera pandemic

The seventh world cholera pandemic began in 1961 and began to rage through Peru in 1991 rapidly spreading throughout South and Central America. There is evidence now to suggest that the eighth pandemic began in Madras in October 1992 and has spread into North-East India and Bangladesh [18]. This organism is not one of the *V. cholerae* 01 strains (classical or El tor biotypes) but a non-01 *V. cholerae* designated 0139 serotype. In the past only the 01 strains of *V. cholerae* have been known to cause epidemics of cholera but molecular genetic analysis of the 0139 serotype has shown that like classical and E1 tor 01 biotypes it produces cholerae toxin [19]. It has been suggested that 0139 is an O-antigen mutant of *V. cholerae* 01 biotype El tor. *V. cholerae* 0139 has been identified in a number of cities in India and Bangladesh and several cases have now been imported into the United Kingdom [20].

New organisms

Microspora

Microsporidiosis has been known to occur in animals for many decades. Its importance as a human infection became apparent during the 1980's with the rise of the HIV/AIDS pandemic. Microsporidiosis produces chronic watery diarrhoea in patients with HIV infection and is clinically indistinguishable from cryptosporidiosis. Within the phylum Microspora, two distinct species are now recognised, *Enterocytozoon bieneusi* and *Septata intestinalis*. These are obligate, intracellular spore forming organisms which predominantly infect the small intestine. The spore is the mechanism by which infection is transmitted and contains a unique structure, the polar tube through which the organism is introduced into the host cell. *E. bieneusi* can be distinguished from *S. intestinalis* as it has a double coiled polar tube where as *Septata* has only a single coil. In addition within the small intestinal epithelial cell, *Septata* is located with a septated parasitophorus vacuole, whereas *E. bieneusi* is free within the cell cytoplasm. Micropridial spores can be detected in faeces using a trichrome stain, although transmission of electron microscopy of the small intestine is generally required to differentiate *E. bieneusi* from *S. intestinalis*. Treatment is with albendazole which generally improves symptoms in patients infected with *E. bieneusi* but often eradicates *Septata intestinalis*.

Cyclospora cayetanensis

Despite the vast numbers of bacteria, viruses and parasites that can cause diarrhoeal disease, new enteropathogens continue to be discovered. In 1989 a previously unidentified organism was found in the stools of 55 immunocompetent foreign visitors in Nepal [21, 22]. The new organism had characteristics of both coccidia and cyanobacteria species and caused a prolonged diarrhoeal illness with anorexia, fatigue and weight loss. A similar organism was identified in Peruvian children during the same period [23] and a further casecontrol study has confirmed the association between chronic diarrhoea and detection of coccidian-like or cyanobacterium-like bodies in the faeces [24]. The organism has been tentatively designated *Cyclospora cayetanensis* and has been identified in an intracellular location in the jejunal epithelium of humans [25]. Exposure to potassium dichromate induces sporulation within 5-13 days following which complete excystation occurs liberating two sporozoites. Electron microscopy has confirmed that the intracellular organelles are characteristic of coccidian organisms [23]. Infection with *Cyclospora* produces shortening of the jejunal villi and results in increased numbers of intraepithelial lymphocytes in the small intestine [25]. Diagnosis relies on microscopic identification of the parasite in faeces or small intestinal aspirate.

A recent double-blind placebo controlled trial in travellers to Nepal with chronic diarrhoea due to *Cyclospora* has shown without doubt that a 7-10 day course of trimethoprim-sulphamethoxazole, two tablets twice daily, will eradicate the infection [26]. In the small proportion of patients in which the infection persists after one week the same treatment should be continued for a further 5-7 days.

Enterhaemorrhagic producing *Escherichia coli* (EHEC)

EHEC were originally identified in 1971 but received little attention until 1982 when serotype 0157: H7 was shown to cause haemorrhagic colitis, usually occuring as foodborne outbreaks related to the ingestion of beef products such as hamburgers [27, 28]. EHEC produce a wide spectrum of disease including asymptomatic infection, mild non-bloody diarrhoea, an illness similar to ulcerative colitis and the haemolyticuraemic syndrome, sometimes with neurological signs. A recent report has suggested that the haemolytic-ureamic syndrome and thrombotic thrombocytopenic purpura may occur in up to 20 % of infected individuals [29]. In the more severe hospitalised cases, mortality may reach 5 %. There is no controlled clinical trial evidence that anti-microbial chemotherapy alters the natural history of infection.

EHEC 0157: H7 and the other EHEC serotypes produce Shiga-like toxin (SLT) I and II. SLT-I has 85 % sequence homology with Shiga toxin and is the more potent of the two. Like Shiga toxin, the SLTs produce their cytotoxic effect by inhibiting protein synthesis of the host cell by binding to the 28S component of ribosomal RNA.

Arcobacter butzleri

An atypical Campylobacter-like organism (CLO) has been identified as a possible cause of recurrent cramping abdominal pain in Italian children [30]. No conventional enteric pathogens were isolated from these children though it was considered likely that the CLO, subsequently identified as *Arcobacter butzleri* by protein electrophoresis and fatty acid analysis, was responsible.

Tropheryma whippelii

Whipple's disease has been recognised to have an infective aetiology for more than eight decades. Bacilli have been identified in macrophages and extracellular locations in the intestine but characterisation has been impossible because of our inability to culture the organism. Using genetic analysis of the 16S-like ribosomal RNA it has been possible to classify this organism and relate it to other bacterial species since the 16S rRNA sequence mutates and makes it useful as an evolutionary clock. According to this phylogenetic analysis, the organism is a gram-positive actinomycete and is not closely related to any known genus [31, 32]. It has been given the name *Tropheryma whippelii*. This work is not only of interest because of its contribution to the classification of the Whipple's bacillus but it has inevitably led to the development of highly specific primers which can be used in a DNA-based polymerase chain reaction assay for detecting the organism in blood and bone marrow. This is an important advance since it may now be possible to screen for this disease without the necessity of obtaining biopsy material from small intestine or brain [33].

New mechanisms

Attachment and adhesins

A key step in the colonisation process for almost all enteropathogens is adherence to the intestinal epithelium [34]. Attachment mechanisms for bacteria and protozoa are often highly specific and mediated by receptor-ligand interactions. Many bacteria such as ETEC utilise adhesins which are lectin or lectin-like molecules which interact with specific sugar moieties on the microvillus membrane. An increasing number of these so-called Colonisation Factor Antigens (CFAs) have been studied extensively in ETEC. More recently, attachment mechanisms of another organism, enteropathogenic *Escherichia coli* (EPEC) have been studied; EPEC is a leading cause of diarrhoea among infants worldwide. The initial phase of EPEC infection involves non-intimate attachment to enterocytes mediated by a bundle-forming pilus which is encoded for by *bfp*A. This gene encodes for a major structural sub-unit of the pilus and is carried on a large plasmid which is common to all EPEC isolates [35]. Following this initial adherence process, the bacterium becomes intimately attached and triggers a major rearrangement of the host cell cytoskeleton, a process known as the *attaching* and *effacing* effect. This process involves activation of host cell tyrosine kinases and liberation of calcium from intracellular stores. This second process is encoded for by a gene cluster located on the EPEC chromosome, designated *eae*A. This gene encodes a 94-kDa membrane protein called *intimin* [36]. This protein shares sequence homology with the invasin proteins of some *Yersinia* sp. A second chromosomal gene, the *eae*B gene, is also necessary for intimate attachment.

To confirm conclusively that these genes encode for important virulence factors, *eae*A deletion mutants have been constructed and administered to healthy volunteers. All volunteers given the wild-type strain developed diarrhoea, whereas only 4 of 11 who received the mutant developed diarrhoea and stool volumes were lower in the mutant group [37]. Thus, the *eae*A gene of EPEC is an important virulence gene for this organism.

EHEC strains also possess an *eae* gene which is thought to be an important virulence factor for EHEC. This has been demonstrated recently in a newborn piglet model of infection by producing an *eae* deletion/insertion mutation in wild-type EHEC 0157: H7 [38]. Without the *eae* gene, EHEC was unable to produce the attaching and effacing lesion in the colonic epithelial cell.

Enterotoxins

Cholera toxin (CT) is the prototype enterotoxin and its mechanism of action has been studied in great detail. Other secretory toxins have also been well characterised including the related *E. coli* heat-labile toxin (LT) and the totally unrelated *E. coli* heat-stable toxin (ST) [34]. Since the discovery of these toxins it has become evident that other bacterial enteropathogens such as *Campylobacter jejuni*, *Salmonella typhimurium*, *Salmonella enteritidis*, *Aeromonas* sp. and *Plesiomonas* sp. also produce LT-like toxins. Other organisms such as *Yersinia enterocolitica* and *Vibrio cholerae* non-01, produce ST-like toxins. However, recent studies suggest that other toxins may also be important in the pathogenesis of cholera. One of the strategies used for the development of attenuated, live oral cholera vaccine strains has been to delete the gene for the A sub-unit of cholera toxin, *ctx*A. One strain, CVD101 in which 94 % of the sequence encoding the A1 peptide of CT had been deleted, continued to produce diarrhoea in the majority of healthy volunteers. Experiments in Ussing chambers have shown that this strain produces a toxin which increases permeability of the small intestinal mucosa by altering the structure of the intercellular tight junction (zonula occludens) [39]. The toxin (zonula occludens toxin, ZOT) is thought to have a molecular weight of between 10-30 kDa, is heat-labile, protease sensitive and has a reversible action *in vitro*. It is not known, however, whether ZOT acts directly on the zonula occludens or is dependant on the production of intracellular messengers. However, a specific receptor for ZOT has been identified in the zonular occludens. The prevalence of ZOT in other strains of *V. cholerae* remains to be established.

By constructing additional plasmids devoid of components of the « core region » of *V. cholerae* it has been possible to identify a third enterotoxin, called accessory cholera enterotoxin (Ace). Ace increases short-circuit current in Ussing chambers and causes fluid secretion in ligated rabbit ileal loops [40]. The predicted protein sequence of Ace shows striking similarity to eukaryotic ion-transporting ATPases, including the product of the cystic fibrosis gene. The gene encoding Ace is located immediately upstream of the genes encoding ZOT and CT. These genes are all located on a dynamic sector of the *V. cholerae* chromosome which can be regarded as a virulence cassette [40]. The development of oral vaccine strains will need to take account of this information if non-diarrhoeaogenic strains are to be developed.

« Enterotoxin-like » activity has been detected in filtered supernatent of stool from *C. parvum*-infected calves [41]. Addition of this supernatent to the mucosal surface of human jejunal mucosal mounted in Ussing chambers produced a chloride-dependent increase in short-circuit current consistent with active chloride iron secretion. The activity was heat-sensitive, calcium-dependent, reversible and saturable. However, it was not possible to determine whether this activity was host or parasite-derived. A similar activity was detected in faecal effluent of AIDS patients with cryptosporidiosis using the Caco-2 cell line [42]. However, the specificity of this observation for *C. parvum* infection could not be determined from these studies as appropriate controls were not included.

Endogenous secretagogues

It is now evident that not all of the secretory effects of CT can be explained simply in terms of activation of adenylate cyclase within enterocytes [34]. 5-hydroxytryptamine (5-HT) is a potent intestinal secretagogue and there is compelling evidence to suggest that it is involved in CT-induced intestinal secretion. Histochemical studies have shown that enterochromaffin cells, a major reservoir 5-HT within the mammalian intestine, are depleted following exposure to CT. Subsequently, it was demonstrated that 5-HT could be found in the intestinal lumen following exposure to CT [43, 44] and that the effects of CT can be substantially reduced in the presence of 5-HT tachyphylaxis in denervated rat small intestine [43]. Furthermore, secretion induced by exogenous 5-HT could be blocked by the neurotoxin, tetrodotoxin, suggesting that a substantial proportion of its effect was mediated by enteric nerves. It was therefore proposed that CT released 5-HT from enterochromaffin cells, which activated 5-HT receptors on afferents of intramural reflex arches controlling intestinal fluid secretion. Further evidence to support this view has been provided by *in vitro* studies in Ussing chambers and *in situ* perfusion of rat small intestine, all of which demonstrate that $5-HT_2$ and probably more importantly, $5-HT_3$ receptor antagonists can markedly reduce and even reverse the secretory state induced by cholera toxins [45-47].

Further support for this concept has been provided by studies in which the myenteric plexus has been ablated by the use of serosal benzalkonium chloride [48]. In segments of intestine in which the myenteric plexus had been destroyed, CT only reduced net fluid absorption whereas in the control non-treated segments there was marked fluid secretion as expected. It was concluded that all afferent fibres in the intramural secretory reflex activated by CT are probably conveyed *via* the myenteric plexus which functions as an integrating centre in the enteric nervous system. The authors also make the point strongly that the Ussing chamber technique using stripped intestinal preparations cannot be used when studying the effects of luminal secretagogues.

Small intestinal epithelial cells receive a rich neural innervation from the sub-mucosal plexus; many nerves contain vasoactive intestinal peptide (VIP) which is thought to be the neurotransmitter. VIP is a potent secretagogue and has been implicated as one of the mediators of CT-induced intestinal secretion. It is proposed that 5-HT released from enterochromaffin cells activate reflex pathways that include cholinergic neurones within the synaptic circuitry and VIPergic motor neurone [34]. VIP released from motor neurones is thought to act on VIP receptors on the basolateral membrane of epithelial cells, inducing secretion and/or inhibiting intestinal absorption.

Other endogenous inflammatory mediators are also involved in the pathogenesis of infective diarrhoea. The pathogenesis of cryptosporidiosis is poorly understood although abnormalities of villus-crypt architecture are recognised to occur in some but not all infected individuals. Recent studies in experimental porcine cryptosporidiosis confirm that villus shortening occurs within 72 hours [49] and intestinal transport studies involving intestinal perfusion and Ussing chambers, confirm that there is reduced fluid and sodium absorption. However, inhibition of prostaglandin synthesis with indomethacin almost completely reversed the impairment in intestinal transport, strongly suggesting that mucosal prostaglandins are involved in the pathophysiology of cryptosporidial diarrhoea [50].

Intestinal anaphylaxis occurs as a result of IgE-mediated immediate hypersensitivity reactions in response to antigens of certain enteropathogens [34]. This process is thought to be particularly important in helminth infections such as those due to *Trichinella spiralis* and *Strongyloides stercoralis* [51]. Studies using specific or relatively specific mediator inhibitors have shown that a variety of mast cell products and neurotransmitters are involved such as histamine, 5-HT, prostaglandins, leukotrienes, platelet activating factor and the neurotransmitter, substance P. A recent study examining the pathogenesis of infection due to the large bowel helminth *Trichuris trichiura* clearly shows that this organism induces an immediate hypersensitivity response in the colon [52], with antigen-induced histamine release being demonstrated in tissue biopsies *in vitro* [53].

Cytotoxins

Many enteropathogens, particularly the invasive organisms, liberate cytotoxins. Shiga toxin produced by *Shigella dysenteriae* type 1 has been extensively characterised with respect to its intestinal receptors and mechanism of action. Recent work on the *Clostridium difficile* toxins A and B has confirmed their importance in the pathogenesis of this infection [54, 55]. Toxin A has both enterotoxin and cytotoxin activity and is a potent neutrophil chemoattractant. Both toxins are lethal when administered parenterally to animals. The genes for both toxins have been cloned and sequenced and are located on the bacterial chromosome. Although toxin A is generally referred to as an enterotoxin, it does not produce intestinal secretion by the classic pathways of CT, LT or ST. Toxin A primarily elicits an inflammatory response with an inflammatory infiltrate in the lamina propria, increased mucosal concentrations of PGE_2 and LTB_4 accompanied by fluid secretion [56]. In addition, there is increased intestinal permeability which appears to be related to disaggregation of actin-containing filaments in the peri-junctional actinomyosin ring. There is increasing evidence to suggest that it is the presence of neutrophils and neutrophil products that mediate these changes. Specific receptors for toxin A have been identified in microvillus membrane and like the Shiga toxin receptor, toxin A receptor is not present in mammalian neonates and this probably explains the absence of disease in human infants infected with *C. difficile* [57].

The large bowel parasite, *Entamoeba histolytica*, also releases a cytotoxin which is a potent pore-forming protein, known as « amoebapore » which produces high conductance ion channels in the target cell resulting in ionic disequilibrium including entry of calcium ions which results rapidly in cell death. Amoebapore is a small 4-8 kDa peptide, with an amphiphilic α-helix and has a structure bearing close homology to melittin, one of the active constituents of Bee venom [58]. Recent work suggests that the pore-forming peptides from nonpathogenic isolates of *E. histolytica* are much less potent than those from pathogenic isolates due to a structural change in the peptide resulting in the shortening of one of the two amphipathic α-helices which are thought to be critical for its pore-forming function [59].

New diagnostic approaches

Since the majority of intestinal infections are self-limiting, one can argue that it is unnecessary to make a specific diagnosis in many cases. This is especially true for the viral diarrhoeas, such as that due to rotavirus or the enteric adenoviruses since knowing the diagnosis does not change management or hasten recovery. Similarly for the vast majority of bacterial diarrhoeas, specific antibiotic therapy is not routinely indicated unless infection is accompanied by severe systemic symptoms with evidence of bacteraemia or septicaemia. However, antibiotic therapy is indicated for dysenteric shigellosis, cholera and *C. difficile* infection and thus it is highly desirable that a microbiological diagnosis is achieved in these situations.

Microscopy

Most bacterial enteropathogens can be detected by routine microbiological culture although special conditions such as prolonged culture are required for the isolation of *Campylobacter jejuni* and *Yersinia enterocolitica*. However, diagnosis of parasitic infection relies heavily on skilled microscopy, often with the use of concentration techniques and special stains. Until recently the diagnosis of microsporidiosis *(Enterocytozoon bieneusi)* has relied on the detection of the parasite by electron microscopy in tissue, usually an intestinal mucosal biopsy specimen. However, a simplified light microscopic technique has been described using formalin-fixed stool specimens and a modified trichrome stain [60]. If tissue specimens are available for examination, then this can provide a valuable diagnostic resource for microsporidiosis, a recent study suggesting that the Warthin-Starry stain is the most effficient way of demonstrating microsporidia in small intestinal biopsies [61].

Faecal antigen ELISA

Faecal microscopy is a laborious and skilled process and thus alternative methodologies have been developed to produce more rapid and objective tests for enteropathogens, particularly parasites. A variety of ELISA's have been developed for the parasites *Giardia lamblia* [62, 63] and *Entamoeba histolytica* [64]. Under experimental laboratory conditions some of these assays have performed well with sensitivities and specificities greater than 90 % but all suffer from the same problem in that the assays produce « false positives ». It is uncertain whether these are in fact true positives, the assays being more sensitive than light microscopy and thus detecting infected individuals by a test that can detect parasites or parasite proteins at a concentration below that which can be resolved by light microscopy. Alternatively, these are true false positives, possibly as a result of cross-reactivity with other luminal antigens. Nevertheless, the assays for *Giardia lamblia* have been commercialised and are now available for routine use [63]. Further controlled evaluation in clinical practice is necessary before their use can be widely recommended.

An alternative approach for the detection of *Entamoeba histolytica* has been to develop an immunoabsorption assay based on the organisms own cysteine proteinase, histolysain [65]. Using a microplate assay, anti-histolysain antibodies are used to capture histolysain from faecal samples, following which the presence of the enzyme is detected using an appropriate substrate and colour reaction. The method has been called Enzymeba and preliminary evaluation has shown it to have an 87.5 % sensitivity and 100 % specificity. Monoclonal antibodies to pathogen-specific epitopes of the galactose adhesin of *E. histolytica* have been used in an ELISA to detect faecal antigen [66]. Preliminary evaluation of the ELISA appears encouraging with specificities and sensitivities of 97 % and 100 %, respectively.

Serology

Detection of specific serum antibodies for the diagnosis of intestinal infection has not found wide acclaim. However, serology has proved useful for the diagnosis of invasive amoebic colitis, for yersiniosis and an IgM assay has been shown to have some value in the diagnosis of acute giardiasis both in adults and children. Serology has also been of value in the diagnosis of certain helminth infections such as schistosomiasis and strongyloidiasis. It can be argued that a serum antibody ELISA is now the screening test of choice for both of these helminth infections. ELISAs have also been developed for the detection of *Echinococcus granulosus* (hydatid disease) which appear to be both highly specific and sensitive [67-69]. Certain refinements have been made in these assays by standardising the hydatid antigen using a synthetic peptide derived from *E. granulosus* recombinant protein [70] or by incorporating a specific monoclonal antibody into a competitive binding assay [71]. Both innovations appear to improve the performance of the assay. An alternative approach has been to use an enzyme-linked immuno-electrotransfer blot test using hydatid fluid as the antigen [69]. Some cross-reactivity was noted in patients with cysticercosis but overall the assay was more specific and more sensitive than the ELISA with which it was compared.

DNA based detection

The genes encoding key virulence factors from many bacterial, viral and parasitic enteropathogens have been cloned and sequenced and it is now possible to develop highly specific DNA probes to detect enteropathogen DNA in faecal specimens, directly or following microbiological culture [72]. Detection of parasites has proved difficult because of the problems in liberating DNA from cysts [73] but these problems will almost certainly be overcome by the use of amplification techniques such as the polymerase chain reaction.

Although as yet these techniques are not widely available in routine laboratories, it seems likely that this will be the case by the end of the decade. DNA based detection techniques, however, will not replace bacterial culture completely because of the need in many instances to obtain information on antibiotic sensitivity of the infective agent.

New treatments

For the majority of self-limiting watery diarrhoeas, oral rehydration therapy is the only treatment that is required. However, there is a continued search for drugs that will reverse or inhibit the secretory process initiated by enterotoxins, such as cholera toxin. Antimicrobial chemotherapy continues to have an important role in the treatment of some bacterial diarrhoeas, particularly those due to invasive micro-organisms; new antibiotic agents are available for bacterial and parasitic infections.

Oral rehydration therapy

Despite the profound secretory state induced by CT and other secretory enterotoxins, substrate-sodium co-transport remains intact and is able to reverse the secretory state for fluid and electrolytes. Similarly, oral rehydration therapy is effective even in rotavirus infection in which there is morphological damage to the small intestine. The ideal composition of oral rehydration solutions (ORS) continues to be discussed with particular controversy surrounding the concentration of sodium and substrate in such preparations [74]. One of the major advances in oral rehydration therapy during the past 5-10 years has been the use of complex carbohydrates such as rice and other cereals; these have improved the effficacy of ORS by reducing the duration of the illness, decreasing the volume of ORS required for rehydration and most importantly by reducing stool volume [75, 76]. This improved efficacy may relate to the increased carbohydrate load that can be delivered as complex carbohydrate [77] although recent studies in model systems suggest that it may relate to the inherently low osmolality of these solutions [78]. Indeed by reducing the osmolality of simple glucose-electrolyte solutions it has been possible to improve water absorption in model systems [79-81] and this improved efficacy has recently been confirmed in two clinical trials [82, 83]. A hypotonic glucose electrolyte formulation has now been endorsed by the European Society for Paediatric Gastroenterology and Nutrition for use in European children [84]. A recent study suggests that in addition to the pro-absorptive effects of rice starch, that rice may also contain an anti-secretory moiety that contributes to its effficacy [85].

Antisecretory therapy

The discovery that 5-HT is involved in CT-mediated intestinal secretion has opened up a therapeutic possibility for the control of secretory diarrhoea. Studies in animal models have shown that prior administration of the $5-HT_3$ receptor antagonists, ondansetron or granisetron either alone or in combination with the $5-HT_2$ antagonist, ketanserin can significantly reduce or even reverse the secretory state induced by CT [45-47]. Recent work confirms that the $5-HT_3$ receptor antagonist, granisetron, can inhibit secretion in a human experimental model of cholera [86]. An alternative approach to controlling intestinal secretion is to inhibit calmodulin, the calcium-binding protein which is important in the control of intracellular calcium concentrations and has a modulatory function on intestinal secretory processes. The calmodulin antagonist, zaldaride maleate, has recently been evaluated in a controlled clinical trials in travellers' diarrhoea and shown to reduce bowel frequency and stool volume without any side-effects [87]. Although these drugs are unlikely to replace oral rehydration therapy in the management of watery diarrhoea, they may have an important contribution to make in reducing fluid and electrolyte losses and thereby simplifying replacement and maintenance therapy.

There is some evidence that bismuth-containing compounds such as bismuth subsalicylate are beneficial in the treatment of watery diarrhoea. The mechanism of how bismuth works in acute diarrhoea is not entirely clear, although there is evidence that it has both antisecretory and antimicrobial activity [88]. A recent placebo controlled study in infants and young children comparing oral rehydration therapy with and without bismuth showed a significant benefit with respect to stool output, duration of hospitalisation and total ORS requirement [89]. The bismuth preparation was given four-hourly which was relatively easy to accomplish in the hospital setting but maybe more difficult in the home. In addition, the major clinical effect of the drug only occurred on the third day and thus treatment would be required to be given for at least three days. The cost implications of this treatment for children in the developing world would be substantial.

Antimicrobial chemotherapy

Although the majority of intestinal infections do not require specific antibiotic therapy, antibiotics are required for the treatment of typhoid fever, dysenteric shigellosis and amoebiasis. Antimicrobials are useful in cholera, giardiasis and in EPEC and *Campylobacter* sp. infections but controversial or at best unknown in non-bacteraemic salmonellosis, yersinosis, *Aeromonas* and *Plesiomonas* sp. infection and cryptosporidiosis [2, 90]. There is, however, compelling evidence that a short course of an antibiotic (1-3 days) will reduce the duration of travellers' diarrhoea with the 4-fluoroquinolones emerging as the drugs of choice [1-3]. A recent study of travellers' diarrhoea in Belize indicates that a single dose of a fluoroquinolone can reduce stool frequency by more than 50 % and the mean duration of illness to less than 24 hours [91]. The decision when to use an antibiotic in travellers' diarrhoea must be made on an individual basis, taking into account the relative risks and benefits. However, ultrashort-term self therapy with an antibiotic would seem to be highly preferable to antimicrobial chemoprophylaxis.

Albendazole is an effective drug for the treatment of helminth infections and in many instances is replacing its widely used predessessor, mebendazole. The therapeutic repertoire of albendazole, however, is extending with further recent encouraging results in the treatment of intra-abdominal hydatid disease. Patients were treated with albendazole for either one month or three months and the results were compared with patients who had not received albendazole prior to surgery. Albendazole treatment for three months resulted in loss of viability in 94 % of cysts compared to 72 % after one month's treatment and 50 % who receive no albendazole treatment. Albendazole treatment has increased total cyst membrane disintegration assessed echographically. The authors conclude that albendazole therapy (10 mg/kg daily) for three months is a suitable alternative to surgery in uncomplicated hydatid liver disease [92].

Albendazole may also be of value in the treatment of microsporidiosis. In an open study of six AIDS patients with microsporidiosis, diarrhoea resolved completely in all within one week of starting treatment and even though relapse occurred in four of these patients between 19-31 days, a second course was successful in controlling the diarrhoea. The drug appeared to have a destructive effect on the parasite and the authors propose that this may be a useful palliative treatment for microsporidial diarrhoea [93].

Albendazole has recently been shown to be of value as « blind therapy » of persistent diarrhoea in patients with HIV/AIDS in Zambia [94]. 173 patients were randomised to receive either albendazole 800 mg twice daily for 14 days or placebo and were then followed at regular intervals for six months. Albendazole significantly reduced the number of days with diarrhoea by 29 % and 26 % of patients achieved a complete remission. Treatment was most effective in patients with Karnofsky score of 50-70 (disability in the mid-range) but did not affect mortality. We had shown previously that microsporidiosis accounted for at least 30 % of cases of persistent diarrhoea in this population and that albendazole-sensitive *Septata intestinalis* was common. We presume that the effficacy of albendazole in this situation relates to its beneficial effects on microsporidiosis, predominantly on *Septata intestinalis*.

Recent *in vitro* studies suggest that albendazole may also have a role in the treatment of giardiasis. The drug has its most profound effects on motility and attachment, which is not surprising since its major therapeutic effects are thought to be related to its inhibitory action on cytoskeletal function [95]. Controlled clinical trials are underway and preliminary results suggest that this drug is both safe and effective for the treatment of giardiasis [96, 97]. It may also find a role in combination therapy for treatment failures in giardiasis. Albendazole therapy may therefore have other useful effects when used in helminth eradication programmes in the community [95].

New approaches to prevention

Ultimately the most effective way to prevent intestinal infection is to avoid entry of the organism into the gastrointestinal tract, which at least theoretically can be achieved by public health measures such as assuring the widespread availability of high quality water, effective sewage control and education to ensure high standards of personal hygiene. These goals are unlikely to be achieved within the next decade and therefore interim strategies are required to minimise the morbidity and mortality associated with these disorders.

Probiotics

Interest continues in the development of innocuous *Lactobacillus* sp. for the prevention of intestinal infection. There is evidence *in vitro* that lactobacilli can inhibit the growth of common enteropathogens [98] although as yet convincing clinical evidence is lacking that these preparations will prevent travellers' diarrhoea and other intestinal infections in humans [99]. We have recently performed a double-blind placebo controlled study of two lactobacilli strains as prophylaxis for traveller's diarrhoea in military personnel beginning a tour of duty in Belize [100]. The acute diarrhoea attack rate in the placebo control group was 23.8 % and this did not differ significantly from either of the two lactobacilli preparations which were given daily for the first 30 days of the tour (lactobacillus LF-KLD 23.8 %, LA 25.7 %). New genetically modified strains of lactobacilli are required to ensure prolonged colonisation of the human intestine.

Chemoprophylaxis

Non antibiotic approaches to chemoprophylaxis such with bismuth subsalicylate have proved effective in preventing travellers' diarrhoea [1-3] although effficacy is considerably less (approximately 65 %) than with antibiotics (greater than 90 %). Nevertheless this approach might be considered in highly susceptible individuals who do not wish to take the risks of antimicrobial chemotherapy [2, 3]. Prophylatic antibiotics are still not widely recommended for general use because it seems inappropriate to put individuals at risk of a life-threatening complication of antibiotic therapy (albeit rare), for what is generally a mild, self-limiting illness. Again there may be situations when short-term antibiotic prophylaxis is appropriate; these options have been discussed in detail in recent reviews [2, 3].

Vaccines

Extensive work continues on the development of vaccines for a variety of enteric infections including typhoid [101, 102] cholera [103] travellers' diarrhoea [104], and a variety of others including rotavirus and shigella. The current strategy has focused on the development of oral, live vaccine strains which have been genetically attenuated, usually by the deletion of important virulance genes such as the gene for CT, *ctx*A. Cholera, rotavirus and typhoid vaccines have received extensive evaluation in the field and will become increasingly available during the next few years [101].

Adapted from: Farthing MJG. Gut infections. In: Pounder RE, ed. *Recent Advances in Gastroenterology 10*. Edinburgh: Churchill Livingstone, 1994: 1-2.

References

1. Farthing MJG. Prevention and treatment of travellers' diarrhoea. *Aliment Pharmacol Ther* 1991; 5: 15-30.
2. Farthing MJG, Du Pont HL, Guandalini S, Keusch GT, Steffen R. Treatment and prevention of travellers' diarrhoea. *Gastroenterol Int* 1992; 5: 162-75.
3. Du Pont HL, Ericsson CD. Prevention and treatment of travellers' diarrhoea. *N Engl J Med* 1993; 328: 1821-7.
4. Farthing MJG. Travellers' diarrhoea. *Gut* 1994; 35: 1-4.
5. Hyams KC, Bourgeois AL, Merrell BR, Rozmajzl P, Escamilla J, Thornton SA, Wasserman GM, Burke A, Echeverria P, Green KY, Kapikian AZ, Woody JN. Diarrheal disease during operation Desert Shield. *N Engl J Med* 1991; 325: 1423-8.
6. Baird-Parker AC. Foodborne salmonellosis. *Lancet* 1990; 336: 1231-5.
7. Telzak EE, Budnick LD, Greenberg MSZ, Blum S, Shayegani M, Benson CE, Schultz S. A nosocomial outbreak of *Salmonella enteritidis* infection due to the consumption of raw eggs. *N Engl J Med* 1990; 323: 394-7.
8. Bandres JC, Mathewson JJ, Dupont HL. Heat susceptibility of bacterial enteropathogens. *Arch Intern Med* 1988; 148: 2261-3.
9. Sheth NK, Wisniewski TR, Franson TR. Survival of enteric pathogens in common beverages: an *in vitro* study. *Am J Gastroenterol* 1988; 83: 658-60.
10. Porter JD, Ragazzoni HP, Buchanon JD, Waskin HA, Juranek DD, Parkin WE. *Giardia* transmission in a swimming pool. *Am J Public Health* 1988; 78: 659-62.

11. Sorvillo FJ, Fujioka K, Nahien B, Tormey MP, Kebabjian R, Mascola L. Swimming-associated cryptosporidiosis. *Am J Public Health* 1992; 82: 742-4.
12. Walker A. Swimming - the hazards of taking a dip. *Br Med J* 1992; 304: 242-5.
13. Balarajan R, Raleigh VS, Yuen P, Wheeler D, Machin D, Cartwright R. Health risks associated with bathing in seawater. *Br Med J* 1991; 303: 1444-5.
14. Elder GH, Hunter PR, Codd GA. Hazardous freshwater cyanobacteria (blue-green algae). *Lancet* 1993; 341: 1519-20.
15. Keene WE, McAnulty JM, Hoesly FC et al. A swimming-associated outbreak of hemorrhagic colitis caused by *Escherichia coli* 0157: 07 and *Shigella sonnei*. *N Engl J Med* 1994; 331: 579-84.
16. Epstein PR, Ford TE, Colwell RR. Marine ecosystems. *Lancet* 1993; 342: 1216-9.
17. Byrd JJ, Huai-Shu XU, Colwell RR. Viable but nonculturable bacteria in drinking water. *Appl Environ Microbiol* 1991; 57: 875-8.
18. ICDDR Cholera Working Group. Large epidemic of cholera-like disease in Bangladesh caused by *Vibrio cholerae* 0139 synonym Bengal. *Lancet* 1993: 342; 387-90.
19. Rivas M, Toma C, Miliwebsky E, Caffer Ml, Galas M, Varela P, Tous M, Bru AM, Binsztein N. Cholera isolates in relation to the « eighth pandemic ». *Lancet* 1993; 342: 925-7.
20. Cheasty T, Rowe B, Said B, Frost J. *Vibrio cholerae* serogroup 0139 in England and Wales. *Br Med J* 1993; 307: 1007.
21. Taylor DN, Houston R, Shlim DR, Bhaibulaya M, Ungar BLP, Echeverria P. Etiology of diarrhoea among travelers and foreign residents in Nepal. *JAMA* 1988; 260: 1245-8.
22. Shlim DR, Cohen MT, Taton M, Rajah R, Long EG, Ungar BL. An algae-like organism associated with an outbreak of prolonged diarrhoea among foreigners in Nepal. *Am J Trop Med Hyg* 1991; 45: 383-9.
23. Ortega YR, Sterling CR, Gilman RH, Cama VA, Diaz F. Cyclospora species - A new protozoan pathogen of humans. *N Engl J Med* 1993; 382: 1308-12.
24. Hoge CW, Shlim DR, Rajah, R, Triplett J, Shear M, Rabold JG, Echeverria P. Epidemiology of diarrhoeal illness associated with coccidian-like organism among travellers and foreign residents in Nepal. *Lancet* 1993; 341: 1175-9.
25. Bendall RP, Lucas S, Moody A, Tovey G, Chiodini PL. Diarrhoea associated with cyanobacterium-like bodies: a new coccidian enteritis of man. *Lancet* 1993; 341: 590-2.
26. Hoge CW, Shlim DR, Ghimire M, Rabold JG, Pandey P, Walch A, Rajah R, Gaudio P, Echeverria P. Placebo-controlled trial of co-trimoxazole for cyclospora infections among travellers and foreign residents in Nepal. *Lancet* 1995; 345: 691.
27. Brook MG, Bannister BA. Verocytotoxin producing *Escherichia coli*. *Br Med J* 1991; 303: 800-1.
28. Burke D, Al Jumaili BJ, Al Mardini H, Record CO. Culture negative cytotoxin positive stools in community acquired diarrhoea. *Gut* 1993; 34: 92-3.
29. Boyce TG, Swerdlow DL, Griffin PM. *Escherichia coli* 0157-H7 and the hemolytic-uremic syndrome. *N Engl J Med* 1995; 33: 364-8.
30. Lior H, Lauwers S. Outbreak of recurrent abdominal cramps associated with *Arcobacter butzleri* in an Italian school. *J Clin Microbiol* 1992; 30: 2335-7.
31. Wilson KH, Blitchington R, Frothingham R, Wilson JAP. Phylogeny of the Whipple's - disease associated bacterium. *Lancet* 1991; 338: 474-5.
32. Relman DA, Schmidt TM, MacDermott RP, Falkow S. Identification of the uncultured bacillus of Whipple's disease. *N Engl J Med* 1992; 327: 293-301.
33. Muller C, Stain C, Burghuber O. *Tropheryma whippelii* in peripheral blood mononuclear cells and cells of pleural effusion. *Lancet* 1993; 341: 701.
34. Farthing MJG. Pathophysiology of infective diarrhoea. *Eur J Gastroenterol Hepatol* 1993; 5: 796-807.

35. Donnenberg MS, Giron JA, Nataro JP, Kaper JB. A plasmid encoded type IV fimbrial gene of enteropathogenic *Escherichia coli* associated with localised adherence. *Mol Microbiol* 1992; 6: 3427-37.
36. Jerse AE, Kaper JB The *eae* gene of enteropathogenic *Escherichia coli* encodes a 94 kilodalton membrane protein, the expression of which is influenced by the EAF plasmid. *Infect Immun* 1991; 59: 4302-9.
37. Donnenberg MS, Tacket CO, James SP, Losonsky G, Nataro JP, Wasserman SS, Kaper JB, Levine MM. Role of the *eae*A gene in experimental enteropathogenic *Escherichia coli* infection. *J Clin Invest* 1993; 92: 1412-7.
38. Donnenberg MS, Tzipori S, McKee ML, O'Brien AD, Alroy J, Kaper JB. The role of *eae* gene in enterohemorragic *Escherichia coli* in intimate attachment *in vitro* and in a porcine model. *J Clin Invest* 1993; 92: 1418-24.
39. Fasano A, Baudry B, Pumplin DW, Wasserman SS, Tall BD, Ketley JM, Kaper JB. Vibrio cholerae produces a second enterotoxin, which affects intestinal tight junctions. *Proc Natl Acad Sci USA* 1991; 88: 5242-6.
40. Trucksis M, Galen JE, Michalski J, Fasano A, Kaper JB. Accessory cholera enterotoxin (Ace), the third toxin of a *Vibrio cholerae* virulence cassette. *Proc Natl Acad Sci USA* 1993; 90: 5267-71.
41. Guarino A *et al*. Enterotoxic effect of stool supernatant of *Cryptosporidium*-infected calves on human jejunum. *Gastroenterology* 1994; 106: 28-34.
42. Guarino A *et al*. Human intestinal cryptospordiosis: secretory diarrhea and enterotoxic activity in Caco-2 cells. *J Infect Dis* 1995; 171: 976-83.
43. Nilsson O, Cassuto J, Larsson PA, Jodal M, Lidberg P, Ahlman H, Dahistrom A, Lundgren O. 5-Hydroxytryptamine and cholera secretion: a histochemical and physiological study in cats. *Gut* 1983; 24: 542-8.
44. Farthing MJG. 5-hydroxytryptamine and 5-hydroxytryptamine-3 receptor antagonists. *Scand J Gastroenterol* (suppl. 188), 1991; 26: 92-100.
45. Beubler E, Horina G. 5-HT_2 and 5-HT_3 receptor subtypes mediate cholera toxin-induced intestinal fluid secretion. *Gastroenterology* 1990; 99: 83-9.
46. Sjoqvist A, Cassuto J, Jodal M, Lundgren O. Actions of serotonin antagonists on cholera toxin-induced intestinal fluid secretion. *Acta Physiol Scand* 1992; 145: 229-37.
47. Mourad FH, O'Donnell LJD, Dias JA, Ogutu E, Farthing MJG. Role of 5-hydroxytryptamine and 5HT type 3 receptors in rat intestinal fluid and electrolyte secretion induced by cholera toxin and *E. coli* heat enterotoxins. *Gut* 1995; 37: 340-5.
48. Jodal M, Holmgren S, Lundgren O, Sjoqvist A. Involvement of the myenteric plexus in the cholera toxin - induced net fluid secretion in the rat small intestine. *Gastroenterology* 1993; 105: 1286-93.
49. Argenzio RA, Liacos JA, Levy ML, Meuten DJ, Lecce JG, Powell DW. Villous atrophy, crypt hyperplasia, cellular infiltration and impaired glucose - NA absorption in enteric cryptosporidiosis of pigs. *Gastroenterology* 1990; 98: 1129-40.
50. Argenzio RA, Lecce J, Powell DW. Prostanoids inhibit intestinal Na Cl absorption in experimental porcine cryptosporidiosis. *Gastroenterology* 1993; 104: 440-7.
51. Harari Y, Russell DA, Castro GA. Anaphylaxis mediated epithelial Cl secretion and parasite rejection in rat intestine. *J Immunol* 1987; 138: 1250-5.
52. MacDonald TT, Choy MY, Spencer J, Richman Pl, Diss T, Hanchard B, Venugopal S, Bundy DAP, Cooper ES. Histopathology and immunochemistry of the caecum in children with the *Trichuris* dysentery syndrome. *J Clin Pathol* 1991; 44: 194-9.
53. Cooper ES, Spencer J, Whyte-Alleng CAM, Cromwell O, Whitney P, Venugopal S, Bundy DAP, Haynes B, MacDonald T. Immediate hypersensitivity in colon of children with chronic *Trichuris trichiura* dysentery. *Lancet* 1991; 338: 1104-7.
54. Lyerly DM, Krivan HC, Wilkins TD. *Clostridium difficile* and toxins. *Clin Microbiol Rev* 1988; 1: 1-18.

55. Torres J, Jennische, Lange S, Lonnroth I. Enterotoxins from *Clostridium difficile*; diarrhoeogenic potency and morphological effects in the rat intestine. *Gut* 1990; 31: 781-5.
56. Moore R, Pothoulakis C, Lamont JT, Carlson S, Madara JL. *Clostridium difficile* toxin A increases intestinal permeability and induces CT secretion. *Am J Physiol* 1990; 259: G165-72.
57. Pothoulakis C, Lamont JT, Eglow R, Gao N, Rubbins JB, Theoharides TC, Dickey BF. Characterisation of rabbit ileal receptors for *Clostridium difficile* toxin A. Evidence for a receptor-coupled G protein. *J Clin Invest* 1991; 88: 119-25.
58. Leippe M, Ebel S, Schoenberger OL, Horstmann RD, Muller-Eberhard HJ. Pore-forming peptide of pathogenic *Entamoeba histolytica*. *Proc Natl Acad Sci USA* 1991; 88: 7659-63.
59. Leippe M, Bahr E, Tannich E, Horstmann RD. Comparison of pore-forming peptides from pathogenic and nonpathogenic *Entamoeba histolytica*. *Mol Biochem Parasitol* 1993; 59: 101-10.
60. Weber R, Bryan RT, Owen RL, Wilcox CM, Gorelkin L, Visvesvara GS. Improved light-microscopical detection of microsporidia spores in stool and duodenal aspirates. *N Engl J Med* 1992; 326: 161-6.
61. Field AS, Hing MC, Milliken ST, MarrioK DJ. Microsporidia in the small intestine of HIV-infected patients. A new diagnostic technique and a new species. *Med J Aust* 1993; 158: 390-4.
62. Rosoff JD, Sanders CA, Sonnad SS, De Lay PR, Hadiey WK, Vincenzi FF, Yajko DM, O'Hanley PD. *J Clin Microbiol* 1989; 27: 1997-2002.
63. Addiss DG, Matthews HM, Stewart JM, Wahlquist SP, Williams RM, Finton RJ, Spencer HC, Juranek DD. Evaluation of a commercially available enzyme-linked immunosorbent assay for *Giardia lamblia* antigen in stool. *J Clin Microbiol*, 1991; 29: 1137-42.
64. Grundy MS, Voller A, Warhurst D. An enzyme-linked immunosorbent assay for the detection of *Entamoeba histolytica* antigens in faecal material. *Trans R Soc Trop Med Hyg* 1987; 81: 627-32.
65. Luaces AL, Pico T, Barrett AJ. The enzymeba test: detection of intestinal *Entamoeba histolytica* infection by immuno-enzymatic detection of histolysain. *Parasitology* 1992; 105: 203-5.
66. Haque R, Kress K, Wood S, Jackson TFHG, Lyeriy D, Wilkins T, Petri WA. Diagnosis of pathogenic *Entamoeba histolytica* infection using a stool ELISA based on monoclonal antibodies to the galactose specific adhesin. *J Infect Dis* 1993; 167: 247-9.
67. Force L, Torres JM, Carrillo A, Busca J. Evaluation of eight serological tests in the diagnosis of human echinococcosis and follow-up. *Clin Infect Dis* 1992; 15: 473-80.
68. Kanwar JR, Kaushik SP, Sawhney IMS, Kamboj MS, Mehta SK, Vinayak VK. Specific antibodies in serum of patients with hydatidosis recognised by immunoblotting. *J Med Microbiol* 1992; 36: 46-51.
69. Verastegui M, Moro P, Guevara A, Rodriguez T, Miranda E, Gilman RH. Enzyme-linked immuno-electrotransfer blot test for diagnosis of human hydatid disease. *J Clin Microbiol* 1992; 30: 1557-61.
70. Chamekh M, Gras-Masse H, Bossus M, Facon B, Dissous C, Tartar A, Capron A. Diagnostic value of a synthetic peptide derived from *Echinococcus granulosus* recombinant protein. *J Clin Invest* 1992; 89: 458-64.
71. Liu D, Lightowlers MW, Rickard MD. Evaluation of a monolonal antibody-based competition ELISA for the diagnosis of human hydatidosis. *Parasitology* 1992; 104: 357-61.
72. Char S, Farthing MJG. DNA probes for diagnosis of enteric infection. *Gut* 1991; 32: 1-3.
73. Butcher PD, Farthing MJG. DNA probes for the faecal diagnosis of *Giardia lamblia* infections in man. *Biochem Soc Trans* 1988; 17: 363-4.
74. Farthing MJG. Oral rehydration therapy. *Aliment Pharmacol Ther* 1994; 64: 477-92.
75. Molla AM, Sarker SA, Hossain M, Molla A, Greenough WB. Rice-powder electrolyte solution as oral therapy in diarrhoea due to *Vibrio cholerae* and *Escherichia coli*. *Lancet* 1982; 1: 1317-9.
76. Molla AM, Molla A, Nath SK, Khatun M. Food-based oral rehydration salt solution for acute childhood diarrhoea. *Lancet* 1989; ii: 429-31.

77. Fayad IM, Hashem M, Duggan C, Refat M, Bakir M, Fontaine O, Santosham M. Comparative efficacy of rice-based and glucose-based oral rehydration salts plus early re-introduction of food. *Lancet* 1993; 342: 772-5.
78. Thillainayagam AV, Carnaby S, Dias JA, Clark ML, Farthing MJG. Evidence of a dominant role for low osmolality in the efficacy of cereal based oral rehydration solutions: studies in a model of secretory diarrhoea. *Gut* 1993; 34: 920-5.
79. Hunt JB, Salim AFM, Thillainayagam AV, Carnaby S, Elliott EJ, Farthing MJG. Water and solute absorption from a new hypotonic oral rehydration solution: evaluation in animal and human perfusion models. *Gut* 1992; 33: 1652-9.
80. Hunt JB, Elliott EJ, Fairclough PD, Clark ML, Farthing MJG. Water and solute absorption from hypotonic glucose-electrolyte solutions in human jejunum. *Gut* 1992; 33: 479-83.
81. Hunt JB, Thillainayagam AV, Carnaby S, Fairclough PD, Clark ML, Farthing MJG. Absorption of a hypotonic oral rehydration solution in a human model of cholera. *Gut* 1994; 35: 211-4.
82. Rautanen T, El-Radhi S, Vesikari T. Clinical experience with a hypotonic oral rehydration solution in acute diarrhoea. *Acta Paediatr* 1993; 82: 52-4.
83. International Study Group on Reduced-osmolality ORS solutions. Multicentre evaluation of reduce-dosmolality oral rehydration salts solution. *Lancet* 1995; 345: 282-5.
84. ESPGAN Working Group. Recommendation for composition of oral rehydration solutions for the children of Europe. *J Paediatr Gastroenterol Nutr* 1992; 14: 113-5.
85. Macleod RJ, Bennett HPJ, Hamilton JR. Inhibition of intestinal secretion by rice. *Lancet* 1995; 346: 90-2.
86. Turvill JL, Mourad FH, Farthing MJG. 5-hydroxytryptamine type 3 (5-HT3) antagonist, granisetron reverses secretion in human cholera model. *Gastroenterology* 1996; 110: A368.
87. Du Pont HL, Ericsson CD, Mathewson JJ, Marani S, Knellwolf-Cousin A-L, Martinez-Sandoval FG. Zaldaride Maleate, an intestinal calmodulin inhibitor in the therapy of travellers' diarrhea. *Gastroenterology* 1993; 104: 709-15.
88. Steffen R. Worldwide efficacy of bismuth subsalicylate in the treatment of travellers' diarrhea. *Rev Infect Dis* 1990; 12 (suppl. 1): 80-6.
89. Figueroa-Quintanilla D, Salazar-Lindo E, Sack RB, Leon-Barua R, Sarabia-Arce S, Campos-Sanchez M, Eyzaguire-Maccan E. A controlled trial of bismuth subsalicylate in infants with acute watery diarrhoeal disease. *N Engl J Med* 1993; 328: 1653-8.
90. Farthing MJG, Katelaris PH, Dias J, Munzer D, Popovic O. Bacterial and parasitic intestinal infections in Europe. *Gastroenterol Int* 1993; 6: 149-66.
91. Salam I, Katelaris P, Leigh-Smith S, Farthing MJG. Randomised trial of single-dose ciprofloxacin for travellers' diarrhoea. *Lancet* 1994; 344: 1537-9.
92. Gil-Grande LA, Rodriguez-Caabeiro F, Prieto JG, Sanchez-Ruano JJ, Brasa C, Aguilar L, Garcia-Hoz F, Casado N, Barcena R, Alvarez Al, Dal-Re R. Randomised controlled trial of efficacy of albendazole in intraabdominal hydatid disease. *Lancet* 1993; 342: 1269-72.
93. Blanshard C, Ellis DS, Tovey DG, Dowell S, Gazzard BG. Treatment of intestinal microsporidiosis with albendazole in patients with AIDS. *AIDS* 1992; 6: 311-3.
94. Kelly P, Lungu F, Keane E, Baggaley R, Kazembe F, Pobee J, Farthing MJG. Albendazole chemotherapy for treatment of diarrhoea in patients with AIDS in Zambia: a randomised double-blind controlled trial. *Br Med J* 1996; 312: 1187-91.
95. Meloni BP, Thompson RCA, Reynoldson JA, Seville P. Albendazole: a more effective antigiardial agent *in vitro* than metronidazole or tinidazole. *Trans R Soc Trop Med Hyg* 1990; 84: 375-9.
96. Dutta AK, Phadke MA, Bagade AC, Joshi V, Gazder A, Biswas TK, Gill HH, Jagota SC. A randomised multicentre study to compare the safety and efficacy of albendazole and metronidazole in the treatment of giardiasis in children. *Indian J Pediatr* 1994; 61: 689-93.
97. Haal A, Nahar Q. Albendazole as a treament for infection with *G. duodenalis* in children in Bangladesh. *Trans R Soc Trop Med Hyg* 1983; 87: 84-6.

98. Itoh K, Freter R. Control of *Escherichia coli* populations by a combination of indigenous *Clostridia* and *Lactobacilli* in gnotobiotic mice and continuous-flow cultures. *Infect Immun* 1989; 57: 559-65.
99. Oksanen PJ, Salminen S, Saxelin M, Hamalainen P, Ihantola-Vormisto A, Muurasniemi-lsoviita L, Nikkari S, Oksanen T, Porsti I, Salminen E. Prevention of travelers' diarrhoea by Lactobacillus. *Ann Med* 1990; 22: 53-6.
100. Katelaris P, Salam I, Farthing MJG. Lactobacilli to prevent travelers' diarrhoea. *N Engl J Med* 1995; 333: 1360-1.
101. Levine MM. Modern vaccines: enteric infections. *Lancet* 1990; 335: 958-61.
102. Simanjuntak CH, Paleologo FP, Punjabi NH, Darmowigoto R, Soeprawoto, Totosudirjo H, Haryanto P, Suprijanto E, Witham ND, Hoffman SL. Oral immunisation against typhoid fever in Indonesia with Ty21a vaccine. *Lancet* 1991; 338: 1055-9.
103. Shharyono, Simanjuntak C, Witham N, Punjabi N, Heppner DG, Losonsky G, Totosudirjo H, Rifai AR, Clemens J, Kaper J, Sorenson K, Cryz S, Levine MM. Safety and immunogenicity of single-dose live oral cholera vaccine CVD 103-HgR in 5-9 year old Indonesian children. *Lancet* 1992; 340: 689-94.
104. Peltola H, Siitonen A, Kyronseppa H, Simula I, Mattila L, Oksanen P, Kataja M, Cadoz M. Prevention of travellers' diarrhoea by oral B-subunit/whole-cell cholera vaccine. *Lancet* 1991; 338: 1285-9.

Gene therapy: basic concepts and applications in gastrointestinal diseases

H.E. Blum, S. Wieland, F. von Weizsäcker

Department of Medicine II, University Hospital, D-79106 Freiburg, Germany

Summary

Genetically, human diseases can be classified into three major categories: (1) monogenetic diseases that are caused by a single gene defect and inherited by the Mendelian rules; (2) complex genetic diseases which are associated with the sequential accumulation of several genetic alterations, only some of which have been identified to date. Several common diseases belong to this category, such as malignancies, diseases of the cardiovascular system, hypertension, arthritis, diabetes mellitus and others; (3) acquired genetic diseases that include infections as well as some malignancies which are associated with the acquisition of genetic alterations during life-time. Based on this genetic classification of diseases, gene therapy involves four concepts: gene substitution for the therapy of monogenetic diseases, gene augmentation for complex genetic diseases, block of gene expression or function for acquired genetic diseases and somatic transgene vaccination for acquired and complex genetic diseases.

Despite exciting prospects of molecular nucleic acid-based therapy of human diseases, including inherited, malignant and infectious gastrointestinal diseases, various delivery, targeting and safety aspects need to be addressed before these concepts will enter clinical practice. Clearly, molecular medicine and gene therapy will increasingly become part of our patient management, complementing existing diagnostic, therapeutic and preventive strategies.

Genetically, human diseases can be classified into three major categories: (1) monogenetic diseases that are caused by a single gene defect, inherited by the Mendelian rules; (2) complex genetic diseases which are associated with several, usually sequential genetic alterations, only some of which have been identified to date; (3) acquired genetic diseases that include infections as well as some malignancies that are associated with the acquisition of genetic alterations during life-time, such as most cases of colorectal cancer (CRC).

Based on this genetic classification of diseases, gene therapy involves four concepts: (1) gene substitution for the therapy of monogenetic diseases, (2) gene augmentation for complex genetic diseases, (3) block of gene expression or function for acquired genetic diseases, and (4) somatic transgene vaccination for acquired and complex genetic diseases. While the concepts of molecular nucleic acid-based therapy of human diseases, including gastrointestinal (GI) diseases, are well defined, various delivery, targeting and safety aspects need to be addressed before gene therapy will enter clinical practice [1, 2]. Clearly, molecular medicine and gene therapy are increasingly part of our patient management, complementing existing diagnostic, therapeutic and preventive strategies.

Basic concepts

Molecular analyses have become a central aspect of biomedical research as well as of clinical medicine during the last few years. The definition of the molecular and genetic basis of many human diseases has led not only to a better understanding of their pathogenesis but has in addition offered new perspectives for their diagnosis, therapy and prevention [3, 4].

Genetically, human diseases can be classified into three major categories [5-8].

(1) Monogenetic diseases that are caused by a single gene defect and inherited by the classical Mendelian rules. There are more than 4,000 monogenetic diseases described. For some of these, the molecular basis has been defined.

(2) Complex genetic diseases which are associated with mutations of several genes, only some of which have been identified to date. Several common human diseases belong to this category, such as malignancies, diseases of the cardiovascular system, hypertension, arthritis, diabetes mellitus and others.

(3) Acquired genetic diseases are infections as well as some malignancies associated with genetic alterations acquired during life-time.

Gene therapy is defined here as the introduction of genetic material into human cells with a therapeutic or preventive advantage to the individual. In the following, we will discuss the basic concepts of gene therapy [5-11], gene delivery and targeting systems as well as some potential therapeutic applications for gastrointestinal (GI) diseases.

Based on the genetic classification of diseases described above, the principle of gene therapy involves four concepts *(Table I)*: gene substitution for the therapy of monogenetic diseases, gene augmentation for complex genetic diseases, block of gene expression or function for acquired genetic diseases and somatic transgene vaccination for acquired and complex genetic diseases.

physiologically not expressed or expressed at therapeutically insufficient levels. This strategy is explored among others for the treatment of malignant diseases. Here, the therapeutic gene product is frequently a cytotoxin that ultimately leads to the elimination of the target cells. Also the introduction of a « suicide gene », such as a gene encoding for herpes simplex virus thymidine kinase (HSV-tk), followed by the administration of aciclovir or ganciclovir, may indirectly result in the killing of the target cell [14].

Block of gene expression or function

For diseases caused by the expression of an acquired gene or the overexpression of an endogenous gene, blocking gene expression can be an effective therapeutic approach. Several strategies can be employed *(Figure 1)*: interfering with the transcription of genes by binding of transcription factors to nucleic acids introduced into or synthesized in the cells (decoy strategy) [15, 16], by binding of single-stranded nucleic acids to double-stranded DNA, forming a triple helix structure [15, 16], hybridization of RNA molecules possessing endonuclease activity (ribozymes) to RNA, resulting in its sequence-specific cleavage [17, 18], block of translation by antisense oligonucleotides [15, 16, 19, 20] and the intracellular synthesis of peptides or proteins, interfering with their normal counterpart (dominant negative mutant strategy) [21].

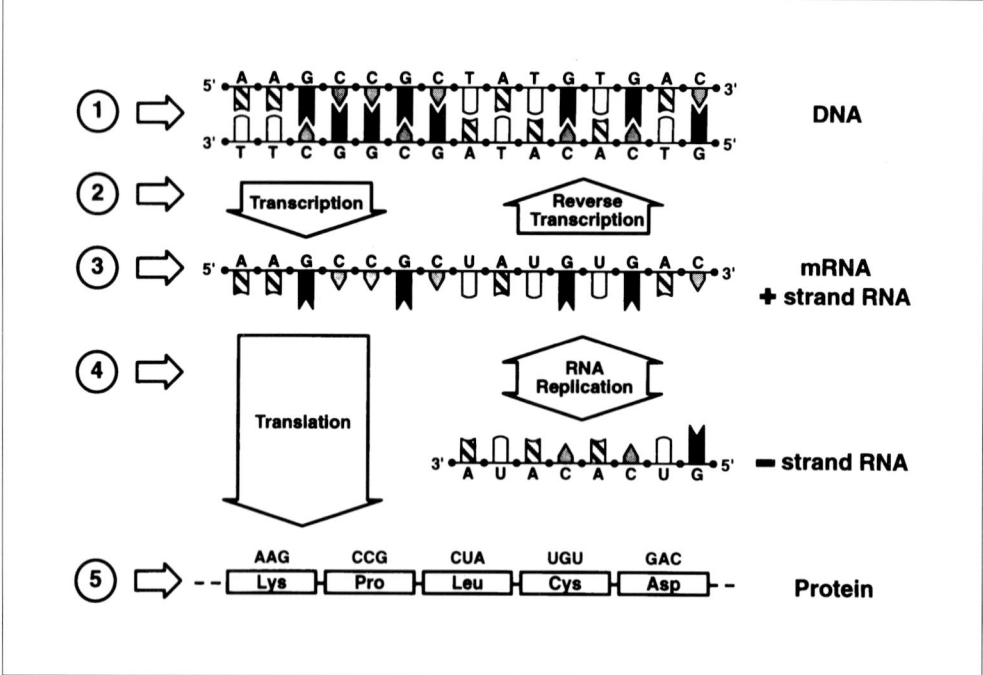

Figure 1. Strategies aimed at blocking gene expression: (1) decoy strategy; (2) anti-gene strategy (triple helix formation); (3) ribozymes; (4) antisense strategy; (5) interfering peptides or proteins.

Somatic transgene vaccination

The direct gene transfer into muscle [22] represents an exciting new development and elegant application of gene therapy [23, 24]. The therapeutic DNA vaccine acts by the intracellular plasmid-derived synthesis of a viral protein which enters the cell's MHC class I pathway [23]. Only proteins that originate within the cell can be processed by MHC class I molecules that carry fragments of the protein to the cell surface. There they stimulate CD8+ cytotoxic T cells, resulting in cell-mediated immunity. In principle, this strategy is applicable to the treatment of acquired genetic diseases, associated with the expression of disease-specific antigens serving as targets for CD8+ cytotoxic T cells.

Gene delivery and targeting

Most important for experimental as well as clinical applications of gene therapy is the efficient transfer (delivery) of nucleic acids to the cells of interest (cellular targeting), within the cells to the correct site (intracellular targeting) as well as the physiological control of gene expression after transduction [1].

Gene transfer

The first step of gene therapy is the reproducible transduction of nucleic acids to target cells. Two basic strategies can be distinguished: viral and non-viral gene transfer systems *(Table III)*.

Table III. Gene therapy: gene transfer methods

Methods	Applications		
Viral	*Ex vivo*	*In vivo*	**Expression**
Retrovirus	+	?	S
Adenovirus	+/-	+	T
Adeno-associated virus (AAV)	+	?	S
Herpesvirus	+/-	+	?
Vacciniavirus	+/-	+	T
Poliovirus	+/-	+	T
Sindbis and other RNA viruses	+/-	+	T
HIV-derived vector	+/-	?	S
Non-viral	*Ex vivo*	*In vivo*	**Expression**
Ligand DNA conjugate	-	+	T
Adenovirus-ligand DNA conjugate	-	+	T
Lipofection	+/-	+	T
Direct DNA injection	-	+	T
Ca-phosphate precipitation	+/-	-	S

Use: + = frequent, +/- = occasional, - = rare. Expression: S = stable; T = transient.

The principle of viral gene transfer systems [25] is the use of genetically modified viruses (viral vectors). The desired gene is cloned into a viral genome made defective by elimination of genes essential for defined aspects of the viral life cycle. The defective recombinant viral genome is transduced into cells which constitutively express the missing viral proteins (« packaging cells »), thereby allowing the coating and export of the defective recombinant viral genome (« packaging »). Packaged defective recombinant viral genomes can infect target cells, followed by the intracellular expression of the therapeutic gene. Due to their defective nature, these genomes cannot replicate on their own. If the defective recombinant viral genome is integrated into the target cell genome, expression of the therapeutic gene can be stable. If the genome is not integrated, expression of the therapeutic gene is transient. For gene therapy a number of viral vectors have been explored *(Table III)*, the best studied vectors being retroviruses, adenoviruses and adeno-associated viruses (AAV).

Retroviruses are RNA viruses which reverse transcribe their genome into DNA. This proviral DNA is stably integrated into the host cell genome and serves as template for transcription into viral RNA and messenger RNA (mRNA). Some retroviruses infect close to 100 % of their target cells, resulting in a highly efficient gene transfer. They infect, however, dividing cells only and have a relatively labile genome, limiting their applications *in vivo*. Different from retroviruses, adenoviruses have a stable genome and infect also non-dividing cells. They do not typically integrate into the host cell genome and, therefore, result in a transient expression of the therapeutic gene only. AAV, on the other hand, can infect non-dividing cells and do integrate into the host cell genome, resulting in stable expression of the therapeutic gene. Also, a recently described human immune deficiency virus (HIV)-derived vector appears to stably transduce non-dividing cells [26].

Apart from viral vectors, a number of non-viral gene transfer systems have been explored *(Table III)*, resulting in the transient expression of the therapeutic gene.

Cellular targeting

A number of different cells have been successfully transduced *ex vivo*: hepatocytes, epithelial cells, keratinocytes, myocytes, fibroblasts, lymphocytes, endothelial cells and a large number of different tumor cells. The selection of the cell type largely depends on the aim of gene therapy. For example, for gene therapy of cystic fibrosis cells of bronchoepithelial origin, for gene therapy of liver diseases hepatocytes are first choices.

Intracellular targeting

Apart from cellular targeting, intracellular targeting and regulation of gene expression are major aspects of gene therapy, especially if stable integration of the therapeutic gene into the target cell genome occurs. Regulation of gene expression is a highly complex and tightly controlled process that depends among others on the correct site of integration into the cellular genome. For example, the expression of beta-globin has to be coordinated with the expression of alpha-globin to yield the biologically active hemoglobin tetramer. Therefore, attempts are made to exactly target the gene of interest to the natural site in the cellular genome *via* homologous recombination (intracellular targeting).

Safety aspects

For experimental and clinical applications of gene therapy, a number of safety issues must be considered [27]. Potential risk are: (1) activation of cellular oncogenes, inactivation of tumor suppressor genes and interference with the cellular DNA mismatch repair system through random integration of the therapeutic gene in the target cell genome; (2) activation of the defective recombinant viral vector through complementation after superinfection of the cell with a wild-type virus; (3) interference of viral gene products with normal functions of the target cell; (4) stimulation of an immune response against the genetically modified target cells; (5) undesired direct cytotoxicity of the therapeutic gene product; (6) contamination of the packaging cell line with wild-type virus, resulting in a productive and potentially lethal infection of the host; (7) mutation of the defective recombinant viral vector *in vivo* with pathogenetic potential in the host. Data available to date demonstrate that these adverse events appear to be extremely rare [9, 10]. Nevertheless, effective and practically implementable control and safety measures are mandatory for experimental and clinical applications of gene therapy.

Gene therapy for gastrointestinal diseases

Based on the genetic classification of diseases described above, the principle of gene therapy of gastrointestinal (GI) diseases involves three concepts: gene substitution for the therapy of monogenetic diseases, gene augmentation or somatic transgene vaccination (STV) for complex genetic diseases and block of gene expression or function as well as STV for acquired genetic diseases. For clinical applications, gene therapy is explored with the aim to either provide novel strategies for diseases for which there is no treatment available or to replace and in some cases complement existing treatment modalities, thereby increasing therapeutic efficacy and/ or reduce adverse events.

Gene substitution

An example for a dominantly inherited monogenetic GI disease is familial adenomatous polyposis (FAP) which is characterized by the progressive development of hundreds of adenomatous colorectal polyps, some of which inevitably progress to colorectal cancer (CRC). The genetic basis of this syndrome in most cases was found to be a germline mutation of the adenomatous polyposis coli (APC) gene. The APC gene encompasses more than 8,500 base pairs and is localized on chromosome 5q21 [28-30]. The APC gene mutations in FAP patients are point mutations as well as small insertions or deletions which frequently result in a truncated APC gene product, due to frameshifts, nonsense mutations or splice site changes, that can be detected at a presymptomatic stage [31].

Functionally, the APC gene can be classified as a tumor suppressor gene. Conceptually, therefore, the delivery early in life of the normal APC gene to the epithelial cells of the colon carrying the mutated APC gene could restore the loss of APC gene function, thereby preventing the development of polyps and CRCs *(Figure 2)*. The clinical applicability of this strategy clearly depends on the availability of an enterocyte-specific and efficient targeting and delivery system (see above).

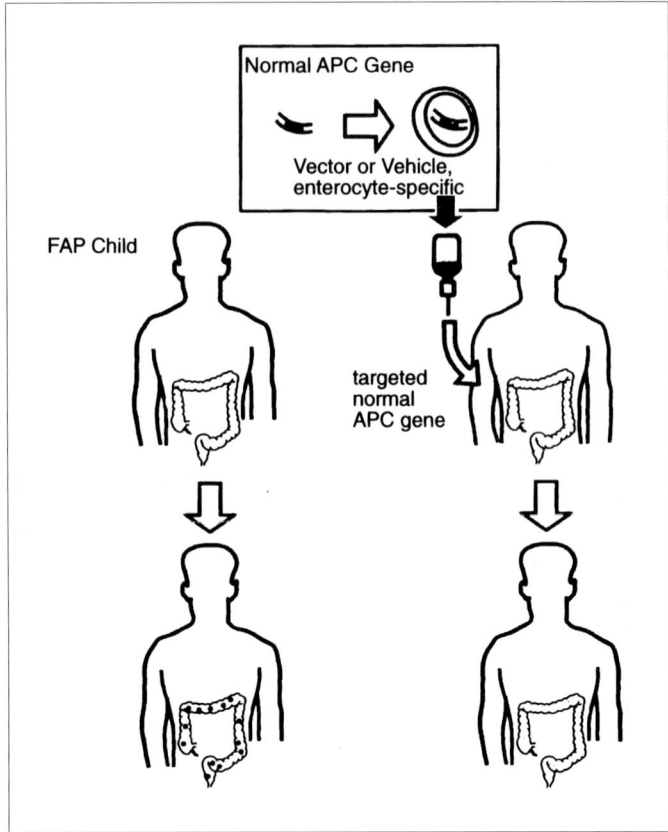

Figure 2. Principle of *in vivo* transduction of the adenomatous polyposis coli (APC) gene into colonic epithelial cells for the prevention of familial adenomatous polyposis (gene substitution).

Gene augmentation

An example for a complex genetic GI disease is CRC. CRC development is a multistep process [32]. In carcinogenesis, the phenotypic changes from adenoma to CRC are paralleled by genetic changes, including mutations in oncogenes, tumor suppressor genes as well as DNA mismatch repair genes [33].

Given the complexity of the genetic changes present in CRCs, the molecular therapeutic strategy is primarily gene augmentation with expression in the tumor of a cytokine, such as interleukin-2 (IL-2) or tumor necrosis factor (TNF), resulting in a local cytotoxic effect [9]. One approach is the *ex vivo* transduction of tumor infiltrating lymphocytes (TILs), isolated from the patient's tumor, with a cytokine gene, such as IL-2 or TNF. After *ex vivo* expansion and reinfusion, the modified TILs find their way to the tumor and express the transduced cytokine gene locally, resulting in local cytotoxicity and regression of the tumor with minimal systemic toxicity *(Figure 3)*.

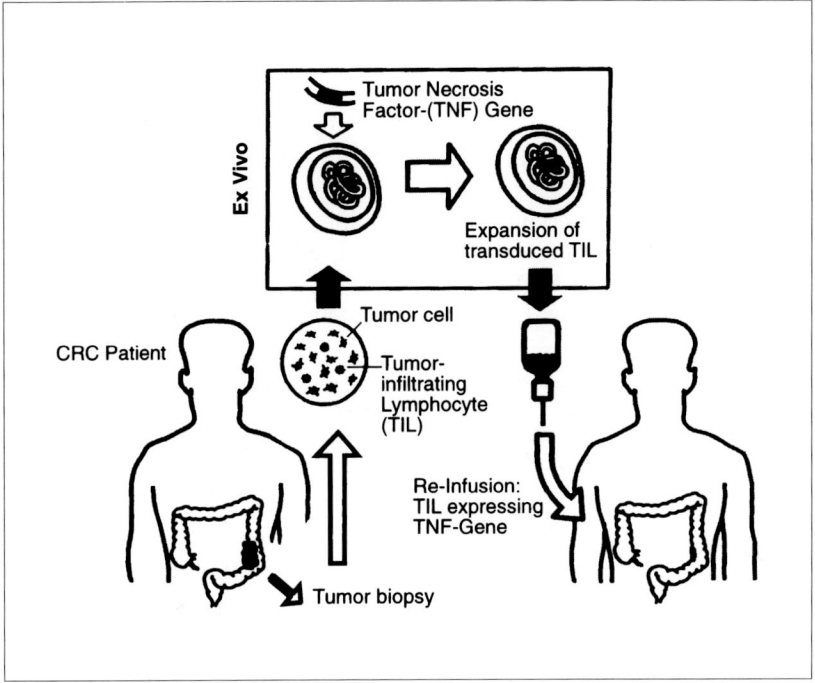

Figure 3. Principle of *ex vivo* transduction of the tumor necrosis factor (TNF) gene into tumor infiltrating lymphocytes (TILs) for the treatment of colorectal cancer (gene augmentation).

Block of gene expression or function

This strategy has been applied to a number of malignant and infectious diseases [15, 16, 19-21, 34-37]. Examples for acquired genetic GI diseases are viral hepatitides as well as most cases of sporadic CRC. The molecular strategies to treat viral hepatitis fall into two main categories: antiviral strategies and elimination of infected cells.

The elimination of infected cells can be achieved, in principle, by immune mechanisms, such as cytotoxic T-cells, by introduction of a « suicide gene », such as a gene encoding for herpes simplex virus thymidine kinase (HSV-tk), followed by the administration of aciclovir or ganciclovir, or by the introduction of genes encoding cytotoxic agents, such as ricin or diphtheria toxin A, that will be activated *via* virus-encoded transactivators only. All these strategies may result in a cytotoxic effect with elimination of the infected cells. To date, the most commonly and successfully used therapeutic strategies are interferon-alpha or -beta which act in part *via* immune modulation, resulting in the immune-mediated elimination of infected hepatocytes.

Antiviral strategies in principle attempt to interfere with one or several aspects of the viral life cycle: attachment of the virus to the cell membrane, internalization and uncoating, viral replication and gene expression, virus assembly and finally virion export. Blocking of viral gene expression or function may efficiently suppress viral infections. Conceptually, molecular or genetic interventions can block viral gene expression at five different levels *(Figure 1)* as well as by novel cytokine-mediated antiviral mechanisms [38].

Decoy strategy

The decoy strategy involves the introduction into cells of oligonucleotides or vectors synthesizing short RNA molecules which are designed to specifically bind to viral or cellular factors, such as transcription or translation factors. The binding of decoys to transcription factors, for example, results in a block of (viral) transcription [15, 16]. The interaction of the decoys, however, with cellular factors, controlling the expression of both cellular and viral genes, may limit this therapeutic approach.

Anti-gene strategy

The anti-gene strategy involves the introduction into cells of oligonucleotides which are designed to bind to double-stranded DNA, resulting in triple helix formation [15, 16], resulting in a reduction of mRNA synthesis [39-41].

Ribozymes

Ribozymes are naturally occurring RNA molecules that catalyze the sequence-specific cleavage of RNA and RNA splicing reactions [17, 18]. Ribozymes that cleave RNA are being developed as inhibitors of gene expression and viral replication. *In vitro* studies have indeed demonstrated that ribozymes can specifically cleave HBV RNA [42]. With respect to hepatitis viruses, however, the *in vivo* application of this strategy has not been successful to date.

Antisense oligonucleotides

Antisense oligonucleotides are designed to specifically bind to RNA or mRNA, resulting in an arrest of RNA replication or mRNA translation *(Figure 4)* [15, 16, 19, 20, 43]. This strategy has been successfully applied *in vitro* to a number of malignant and viral diseases, including HBV infection *(Figure 5)* [36, 44, 45] and HCV infection [46-48]. In addition, studies in the duck hepatitis B virus (DHBV) model of HBV infection demonstrated the principle of the *in vivo* applicability of this approach [49].

Interfering peptides or proteins

The intracellular synthesis of interfering peptides or proteins, including antibodies, is aimed at the specific interference with the assembly or function of (viral) structural or non-structural proteins and represents a type of intracellular immunization [50]. This approach is being explored, among others, for the inhibition of HBV core particle production using modified viral core proteins [51-53].

Cytokine-mediated antiviral mechanisms

Recent evidence in a transgenic mouse model suggests that virus-specific cytotoxic T cells (CTLs) can abolish HBV gene expression and replication in liver cells without hepatocyte

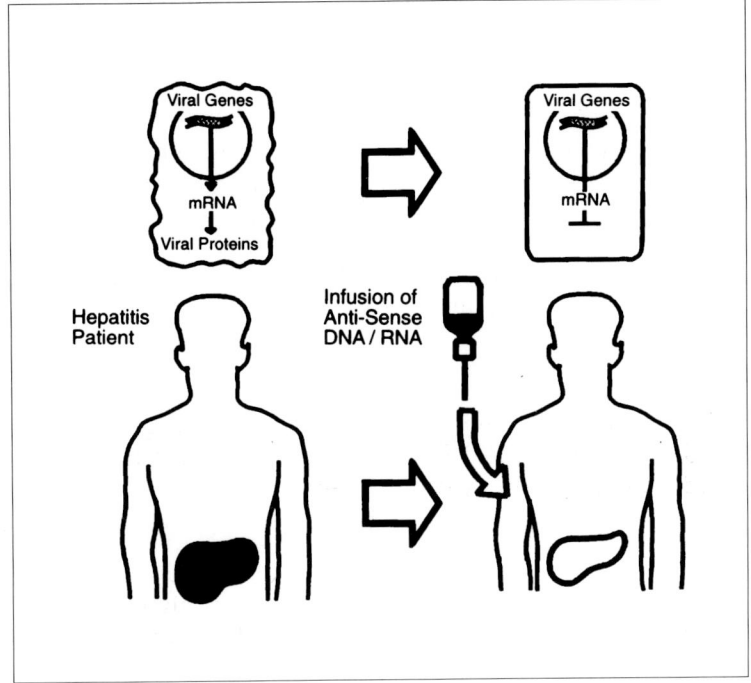

Figure 4. Principle of *in vivo* therapy of viral hepatitis by antisense oligonucleotides (block of gene expression).

killing [38]. This antiviral effect is mediated through interferon gamma (IFN-gamma) and tumor necrosis factor alpha (TNF-alpha) secreted by the CTLs or by the antigen-nonspecific macrophages and T cells that they activate following antigen recognition [38, 54]. These cytokines appear to act *via* elimination of nucleocapsid particles and replicating viral genomes as well as through destabilization of viral RNA [38]. IFN-alpha and -beta as well as interleukin-2 (IL-2) appear to act, at least in part, *via* the same pathways [55, 56]. Gene therapy aimed at the local expression of IFN-gamma or TNF-alpha, therefore, may prove to be an effective antiviral strategy. Therapeutic DNA vaccination (see below) possibly also acts *via* cytokine-mediated intracellular inactivation of viral replication and gene expression [38].

The molecular strategies presently being explored to block viral gene expression at different levels still face a number of problems. Apart from the optimal design of such oligonucleotides or DNA constructs, a major problem is the stability of these therapeutic nucleic acids *in vivo* as well as their specific cellular and intracellular targeting (see above). Viral and non-viral vectors, including liposomes [57] or immunoliposomes [58] and recombinant chylomicrons [59], are being investigated and should allow the specific delivery of antiviral molecules to infected cells, thereby improving therapeutic efficacy and reducing extrahepatic side-effects.

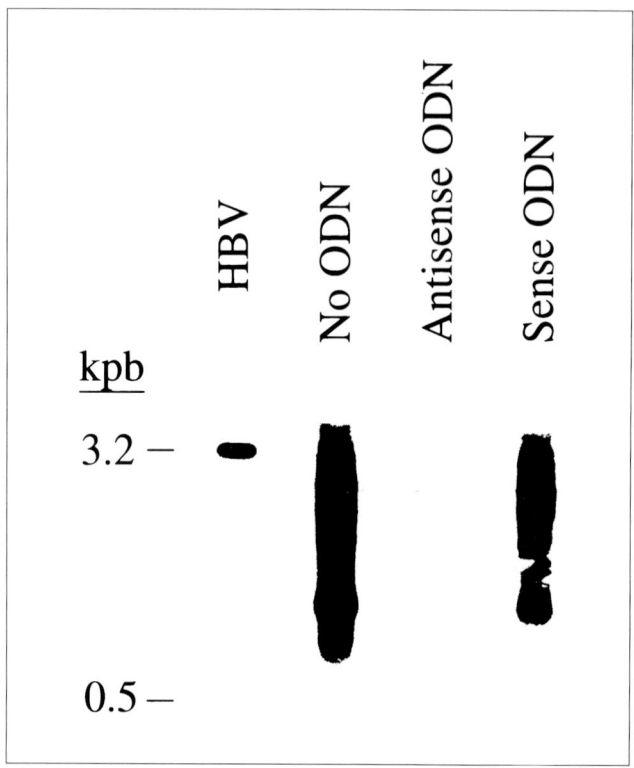

Figure 5. Inhibition of hepatitis B virus (HBV) replication *in vitro* by antisense oligonucleotides (block of gene expression). Southern blot analysis of DNA isolated from HBV DNA transfected hepatoma cells [45].

Somatic transgene vaccination

An elegant and innovative application of gene therapy is the manipulation of the immune system by introduction of expression vectors into muscle cells, resulting in long lasting cellular and humoral immune responses [22-24, 60].

DNA-based prophylactic vaccination against HBV infection, for example, is possible by intramuscular introduction of a plasmid expressing hepatitis B surface antigen (HBsAg). HBsAg is taken up by cells *via* phagocytosis or endocytosis, processed through the major histocompatibility complex (MHC) class II system and primarily stimulates an antibody response through CD4+ helper T cells with the production of anti-HBs [23, 24, 61, 62].

By contrast, the therapeutic DNA vaccine acts by the intracellular plasmid-derived synthesis of a viral protein which enters the cell MHC class I pathway, [23]. Therapeutic DNA vaccination has been experimentally explored already for HBV infection [63-65] as well as for HCV infection [66, 67] and holds great promise as an effective molecular therapy for these viral diseases. Further, suppressive vaccination with DNA encoding a variable region gene of the T-cell receptor has recently been shown to prevent autoimmune encephalomyelitis, making this approach attractive for the treatment of Th1 mediated diseases, such as multiple sclerosis, juvenile diabetes or rheumatoid arthritis [68].

References

1. Crystal RG. Transfer of genes to humans: early lessons and obstacles to success. *Science* 1995; 270: 404-10.
2. Friedmann T. Human gene therapy - an immature genie, but certainly out of the bottle. *Nature Med* 1996; 2: 144-7.
3. Blum HE, von Weizsäcker F, Walter E. Gentechnologie: Medizinische Bedeutung. *Dtsch Med Wschr* 1993; 118: 629-33.
4. Blum HE, von Weizsäcker F, Walter E. Grundlagen der Gentechnologie. *Dtsch Med Wschr* 1993; 118: 589-92.
5. Anderson WF. Human gene therapy. *Science* 1992; 256: 808-13.
6. Friedmann T. Progress toward human gene therapy. *Science* 1989; 244: 1275-81.
7. Gutierrez AA, Lemoine NR, Sikora K. Gene therapy for cancer. *Lancet* 1992; 339: 715-21.
8. Miller AD. Human gene therapy comes of age. *Nature* 1992; 357: 455-60.
9. Morgan RA, Anderson WF. Human gene therapy. *Annu Rev Biochem* 1993; 62: 191-217.
10. Mulligan RC. The basic science of gene therapy. *Science* 1993; 260: 926-32.
11. Rosenberg SA. Gene therapy for cancer. *JAMA* 1992; 268: 2416-9.
12. Sarver N, Cairns S. Ribozyme trans-splicing and RNA tagging: following the messenger. *Nature Med* 1996; 2: 641-2.
13. Jones JT, Lee SW, Sullenger BA. Tagging ribozyme reaction sites to follow *trans*-splicing in mammalian cells. *Nature Med* 1996; 2: 643-8.
14. Caruso M, Panis Y, Gagandeep S, Houssin D, Salzmann JL, Klatzmann D. Regression of established macroscopic liver metastases after *in situ* transduction of a suicide gene. *Proc Natl Acad Sci USA* 1993; 90: 7024-8.
15. Helene C. Rational design of sequence-specific oncogene inhibitors based on antisense and antigene oligonucleotides. *Eur J Cancer* 1991; 27: 1466-71.
16. Helene C, Toulme JJ. Specific regulation of gene expression by antisense, sense and antigene nucleic acids. *Biochim Biophys Acta* 1990; 1049: 99-125.
17. Haseloff J, Gerlach WL. Simple RNA enzymes with new and highly specific endoribonuclease activities. *Nature* 1988; 334: 585-91.
18. Thompson JD, Macejak D, Couture L, Stinchcomb DT. Ribozymes in gene therapy. *Nature Med* 1995; 1: 277-8.
19. Calabretta B. Inhibition of protooncogene expression by antisense oligodeoxynucleotides: biological and therapeutic implications. *Cancer Res* 1991; 51: 4505-10.
20. Tseng BY, Brown KD. Antisense oligonucleotide technology in the development of cancer therapeutics. *Cancer Gene Ther* 1994; 1: 65-71.
21. Herschkowitz I. Functional inactivation of genes by dominant negative mutations. *Nature* 1987; 329: 219-22.
22. Blau HM, Springer ML. Muscle mediated gene therapy. *N Engl J Med* 1995; 333: 1554-6.
23. McDonnell WM, Askari FK. DNA vaccines. *N Engl J Med* 1996; 334: 42-5.
24. Pardoll DM, Beckerleg AM. Exposing the immunology of naked DNA vaccines. *Immunity* 1995; 3: 165-9.
25. Jolly D. Viral vector systems for gene therapy. *Cancer Gene Ther* 1994; 1: 51-64.
26. Naldini L, Blömer U, Gallay P, Ory D, Mulligan R, Gage F, Verma IM, Trono D. *In vivo* gene delivery and stable transduction of nondividing cells by a lentiviral vector. *Science* 1996; 272: 263-7.

27. Koch-Brandt C. *Gentransfer. Prinzipien, Experimente, Anwendung bei Säugern.* Stuttgart, New York: Georg Thieme Verlag, 1993.
28. Groden J et al. Identification and characterization of the familial adenomatous polyposis coli gene. *Cell* 1991; 66: 589-600.
29. Kinzler KW et al. Identification of FAP locus genes from chromosome 5q21. *Science* 1991; 253: 661-5.
30. Nishisho I et al. Mutations of chromosome 5q21 genes in FAP and colorectal cancer patients. *Science* 1991; 253: 665-9.
31. Powell SM et al. Molecular diagnosis of familial adenomatous polyposis. *N Engl J Med* 1993; 329: 1982-7.
32. Fearon ER, Vogelstein B. A genetic model for colorectal tumorigenesis. *Cell* 1990; 61: 759-67.
33. Toribara NW, Sleisenger MH. Screening for colorectal cancer. *N Engl J Med* 1995; 332: 861-7.
34. Chatter JS, Johnson PR, Wong KK. Dual-target inhibition of HIV-1 *in vitro* by means of an adeno-associated antisense vector. *Science* 1992; 258: 1485-8.
35. Trono D, Feinberg MB, Baltimore D. HIV-1 gag mutants can dominantly interfere with the replication of the wild type virus. *Cell* 1992; 59: 113-20.
36. Wu GY, Wu CH. Specific inhibition of hepatitis B viral gene expression *in vitro* by targeted antisense oligonucleotides. *J Biol Chem* 1992; 267: 12436-9.
37. Monia BP, Johnston JF, Geiger T, Muller M, Fabbro D. Antitumor activity of a phosphorothioate antisense oligodeoxynucleotide targeted against C-*raf* kinase. *Nature Med* 1996; 2: 668-75.
38. Guidotti LG, Ishikawa T, Hobbs MV, Matzke B, Schreiber R, Chisari FV. Intracellular inactivation of the hepatitis B virus by cytotoxic T lymphocytes. *Immunity* 1996; 4: 25-36.
39. Strobel SA, Dervan PB. Site specific cleavage of a yeast chromosome by oligonucleotide directed triple helix formation. *Science* 1990; 249: 73-5.
40. Postel EH, Flint SJ, Kessler DJ, Hogan ME. Evidence that a triplex forming oligodeoxyribonucleotide binds to the c-myc promoter in HeLa cells, thereby reducing c-myc mRNA levels. *Proc Natl Acad Sci USA* 1991; 88: 8227-31.
41. Duval VG, Thuong NT, Helene C. Specific inhibition of transcription by triple helix-forming oligonucleotides. *Proc Natl Acad Sci USA* 1992; 89: 504-8.
42. von Weizsäcker F, Blum HE, Wands JR. Cleavage of hepatitis B virus RNA by three ribozymes transcribed from a single DNA template. *Biochem Biophys Res Commun* 1992; 189: 743-8.
43. Wagner RW. Gene inhibition using antisense oligodeoxynucleotides. *Nature* 1994; 372: 333-5.
44. Goodarzi G, Gross SC, Tewari A, Watabe K. Antisense oligodeoxyribonucleotides inhibit the expression of the gene for hepatitis B virus surface antigen. *J Gen Virol* 1990; 71: 3021-5.
45. Blum HE, Galun E, Weizsäcker F, Wands JR. Inhibition of hepatitis B virus by antisense oligodeoxynucleotides (letter). *Lancet* 1991; 337: 1230.
46. Wakita T, Wands JR. Specific inhibition of hepatitis C virus expression by antisense oligodeoxynucleotides. *In vitro* model for selection of target sequence. *J Biol Chem* 1994; 269: 14205-10.
47. Mizutani T, Kato N, Hirota M, Sugiyama K, Murakami A, Shimotohno K. Inhibition of hepatitis C virus replication by antisense oligonucleotide in culture cells. *Biochem Biophys Res Commun* 1995; 212: 906-11.
48. Alt M, Renz R, Hofschneider P H, Paumgartner G, Caselmann WH. Specific inhibition of hepatitis C viral gene expression by antisense phosphorothioate oligodeoxynucleotides. *Hepatology* 1995; 22: 707-17.
49. Offensperger WB, Offensperger S, Walter E, Teubner K, Igloi G, Blum HE, Gerok W. *In vivo* inhibition of duck hepatitis B virus replication and gene expression by phosphorothioate modified antisense oligodeoxynucleotides. *EMBO J* 1993; 12: 1257-62.
50. Baltimore D. Intercellular immunization. *Nature* 1988; 325: 395-6.
51. Delaney MA, Goyal S, Seeger C. In: Hollinger FB, Lemon SM and Margolis H, eds. *Viral hepatitis and liver disease.* Baltimore, Maryland: Williams & Wilkins, 1991; 667-8.

52. Scaglioni PP, Melegari M, Wands JR. Characterization of hepatitis B virus core mutants that inhibit viral replication. *Virology* 1994; 205: 112-20.
53. von Weizsäcker F, Wieland S, Blum HE. Inhibition of viral replication by genetically engineered mutants of the duck hepatitis B virus core protein. *Hepatology* 1996; 24: in press.
54. Guidotti LG, Ando K, Hobbs MV, Ishikawa T, Runkel L, Schreiber RD, Chisari FV. Cytotoxic T lymphocytes inhibit hepatitis B virus gene expression by a noncytolytic mechanism in transgenic mice. *Proc Natl Acad Sci USA* 1994; 91: 3764-8.
55. Guilhot S, Guidotti LG, Chisari FV. Interleukin-2 downregulates hepatitis B virus gene expression in transgenic mice by a posttranscriptional mechanism. *J Virol* 1993; 67: 7444-9.
56. Guidotti LG, Guilhot S, Chisari FV. Interleukin-2 and alpha/beta interferon down-regulate hepatitis B virus gene expression *in vivo* by tumor necrosis factor-dependent and -independent pathways. *J Virol* 1994; 68: 1265-70.
57. Rose JK, Buonocore L, Whitt MA. A new cationic liposome reagent mediating nearly quantitative transfection of animal cells. *Biotechniques* 1991; 10: 520-5.
58. Kalvakolanu DV, Abraham A. Preparation and characterization of immunoliposomes for targeting of antiviral agents. *Biotechniques* 1991; 11: 218-22.
59. Rensen PCN, Vandijk MCM, Havenaar EC, Bijstersbosch MK, Kruijt JK, Vanberkel TJC. Selective liver targeting of antivirals by recombinant chylomicrons: a new therapeutic approach to hepatitis B. *Nature Med* 1995; 1: 221-5.
60. Kumar V, Sercarz E. Genetic vaccination: the advantages of going naked. *Nature Med* 1996; 2: 857-9.
61. Davis HL, Michel ML, Whalen RG. DNA-based immunization induces continuous secretion of hepatitis B surface antigen and high levels of circulating antibody. *Hum Mol Genet* 1993; 2: 1847-51.
62. Davis HL, McCluskie MJ, Gerin JL, Purcell RH. DNA vaccine for hepatitis B: evidence for immunogenicity in chimpanzees and comparison with other vaccines. *Proc Natl Acad Sci USA* 1996; 93: 7213-8.
63. Schirmbeck R, Bohm W, Ando K, Chisari FV, Reimann J. Nucleic acid vaccination primes hepatitis B virus surface antigen specific cytotoxic T lymphocytes in nonresponder mice. *J Virol* 1995; 69: 5929-34.
64. Vitiello A *et al*. Development of a lipopeptide based therapeutic vaccine to treat chronic HBV infection. I. Induction of a primary cytotoxic T lymphocyte response in humans. *J Clin Invest* 1995; 95: 341-9.
65. Kuhöber A, Pudollek HP, Reifenberg K, Chisari FV, Schlicht HJ, Reimann J, Schirmbeck R. DNA immunization induces antibody and cytotoxic T cell responses to hepatitis B core antigen in H-2b mice. *J Immunol* 1996; 156: 3687-95.
66. Lagging LM, Meyer K, Hoft D, Houghton M, Belshe RB, Ray R. Immune responses to plasmid DNA encoding the hepatitis C virus core protein. *J Virol* 1995; 69: 5859-63.
67. Major ME, Vitvitski L, Mink MA, Schleef M, Whalen RG, Trepo C, Inchauspe G. DNA based immunization with chimeric vectors for the induction of immune responses against the hepatitis C virus nucleocapsid. *J Virol* 1995; 69: 5798-805.
68. Waisman A *et al*. Suppressive vaccination with DNA encoding a variable region gene of the T-cell receptor prevents autoimmune encephalomyelitis and activates Th2 immunity. *Nature Med* 1996; 2: 899-905.

Vaccinating against *Helicobacter pylori* infections: reality and perspectives

A. Labigne, R. Ferrero

Unité de Pathogénie Bactérienne des Muqueuses, INSERM U 389, Institut Pasteur, 25, rue du Docteur-Roux, 75724 Paris Cedex 15, France

Summary

The high prevalence of Helicobacter pylori *infections, the severity of certain associated pathologies (duodenal ulcers, lymphoma, gastric carcinoma) and the predictable gradual emergence of resistance to the antibiotics currently used are factors that have encouraged the development of a vaccine approach to* H. pylori *infections. Studies to date have demonstrated that it is possible to protect animals (mice, ferrets, cats) against* Helicobacter *infection by immunisation via the oral-gastric route using crude extracts of bacterial antigens combined with an adjuvant known to stimulate a mucosal immune response. More recently, better defined* H. pylori *antigens such as the urease subunits, the HspA protein or the VacA cytotoxin, have been identified as possible components of a recombinant subunit vaccine. Progress achieved over the last few years in animal models leads us to expect that a prophylactic and/or therapeutic vaccine will be a reality in the first decade of the 21st century.*

Helicobacter pylori is implicated in the origin of gastro-duodenal inflammatory diseases; it is the major etiologic agent of chronic gastritis, and is also responsible for the evolution from chronic gastritis to ulcers, or to gastric atrophy, the precursor of adenocarcinoma of the stomach. Peptic ulcer disease affects about 10% of the population in Western countries, and is now unanimously recognized as an infectious disease. As for any infectious disease, it was therefore legitimate to seek to develop a vaccine approach to prevent or eradicate *H. pylori* infections.

Until 1993, the very idea of a vaccine against *H. pylori* infections was the object of considerable skepticism and numerous polemics due to the fact that *H. pylori* infection was known to go hand in hand with a strong host immune response (both local and systemic), and that this response had no effect on the clearance of bacteria from the gastric mucosa. It was thus likely that to be successful, a vaccine approach should aim at targeting the bacterial antigens involved in the early stages of colonization of the gastric mucosa, and specifically stimulate a local immune response in the gastric mucosa.

Identification of bacterial antigens involved in the early stages of colonization of the gastric mucosa

All bacteria of the *Helicobacter* genus that colonize the gastric mucosa of mammals produce a urease enzyme that exhibits unique features; it is composed of two subunits (UreA and UreB), instead of the three that are usually found in other bacterial ureases, it is an abundant enzyme accounting for up to 6% of the protein content of *Helicobacter pylori*, and it is an extracellular enzyme. This metallo-enzyme, which is active in the presence of nickel ions, was initially suspected to be one of the key enzymes that confers the ability of the bacteria to survive and colonize the gastric mucosa. This was indeed confirmed with the identification of seven urease genes in *H. pylori* [1, 2] and also in *H. felis* [3], a bacterium that naturally colonizes the gastric mucosa of cats, and experimentally, of the mouse. The construction of mutants of *H. pylori* in which each of the seven genes was precisely inactivated by reverse genetics (creating isogenic mutants) [4], confirmed that each of the seven genes were all involved in the expression of a catalytically active urease. Two of them (ureA and ureB) are structural genes governing the synthesis of the two urease subunits, the others are accessory genes involved in the activation of the apoenzyme into a catalytically active molecule (ureI, ureE, ureF, ureG, and ureH). Such non-ureolytic isogenic mutants of *H. pylori* were used to infect gnotobiotic piglets [5], but were not able to colonize the gastric mucosa of these animals, proving that urease plays a vital role in colonization, enabling the survival of the bacteria.

Linked to the characterization of this were the genetic and molecular studies of *H. pylori* which led to the identification of a second antigen with characteristics unique in the bacterial world. This antigen, called HspA, is a homologue of the *E. coli* GroES protein, although it has an unusual structure for such a homologue [6]; its C-terminal extremity has a 27 amino acid sequence containing a series of histidines and cysteines totally absent from the other bacterial GroES proteins. This C-terminal sequence has a high and specific affinity for nickel ions and participates in the enhancement of urease activity in *E. coli*, suggesting that the HspA protein of *H. pylori* plays an important role in urease activity. The determination of the nucleotide sequence of the HspA gene in 35 different clinical isolates has revealed that the sequence is highly conserved from one clinical strain to another.

These genetic studies have therefore enabled us to identify three major extracellular antigens that are essential for the successful bacterial colonization of the gastric mucosa. These antigens were cloned into different expression vectors, either in their native state or fused, and enabled us to produce UreA, UreB, or HspA on a large scale.

Stimulation of the immune response of the gastric mucosa protects against *Helicobacter* infections in murine models

In 1993 two teams, Hazell and Lee [7] in Australia and Czinn and Nedrud [8] in the United States, used a mouse model colonized by *Helicobacter felis*, a bacterium similar to *H. pylori*, to demonstrate that it was possible to protect against colonization of the gastric mucosa by *Helicobacter* bacteria. These immunizations were carried out *via* the oralgastric route using sonicated *H. felis* preparations administered together with cholera toxin. In contrast to the numerous unsuccessful attempts to immunize by intravenous or parenteral routes, these results demonstrate how important it is to stimulate the mucosal immune system to protect against *Helicobacter*. More recently (1994), the same Australian team demonstrated that it was possible to eradicate *Helicobacter* from the gastric mucosa of mice by oral administration of the same sonicate extract used as vaccinal preparation [9].

These ground-breaking experiments demonstrated the feasibility of a vaccine approach, both for prophylactic and therapeutic uses, to eradicate *Helicobacter* infections. However, a crude extract of this type cannot be used as a vaccine due to the presence of endotoxin and other potential bacterial toxins. Thus, the identification of protective components in these complex mixtures of antigens was necessary.

Another major breakthrough occurred in 1995, with the development of conventional mouse models colonized by *H. pylori* strains freshly isolated from human biopsies [10, 11]. Although these models appear promising, it remains unclear whether the colonization persists, whether chronic gastritis appears, and whether the various pathologies associated with *H. pylori* in humans will develop in mice.

From the crude bacterial extract to the recombinant sub-unit vaccine

The urease sub-units were rapidly recognized as putative antigen candidates for inclusion in a prophylactic recombinant sub-unit vaccine. This choice was motivated by the fact that the genetic analyses that had been performed on the urease gene cluster permitted the production of large amount of recombinant antigens, and second by the intrinsic properties of these antigens, namely their ubiguity, their lack of antigenic variation and that they are essential proteins.

The first demonstration of immune protection of mice after immunization with native *H. pylori* urease followed by recombinant urease sub-units using the *H. felis* mouse model were reported by Michetti *et al.* [12]. Our group [13] and that of OraVax [14] have subsequently confirmed the protective role of urease sub-units in the mouse *H. felis* model. More recently, investigators at Biocine [15], Cuenca *et al.* [16], confirmed these findings in the *H. pyloris* mouse model and the *H. mustelae* ferret model, respectively.

In protection studies conducted by Ferrero et al. [13], the fusion proteins MalE-UreA and MalE-UreB of *H. pylori* (heterologous antigens), of *H. felis* (homologous antigens) and the MalE-HspA of *H. pylori* were used. The protective effects of homologous recombinant proteins were compared to that of heterologous proteins. These were also compared to a mixture of antigens derived from the sonicated *H. felis* preparation. Neither the sub-unit UreA of *H. pylori* nor that of *H. felis* had any protective effect. UreB from both *H. felis* and *H. pylori* had protective effects; as expected, homologous antigen had the greater protective effect.

HspA has the same protective potential in mice as UreB when used as a protein fused to the maltose binding protein [17]. More interestingly, the combination of HspA in the presence of a second antigen such as UreB appeared to be synergistic; indeed, when MBP-HspA was administered together with MBP-UreB, they induced a level of protection equivalent to that obtained by immunization of mice with a mixture of sonicated antigens [17].

The results published to date thus identify three recombinant polypeptides that have a protective effect:

(1) the sub-unit UreB which, when administrated alone, confers 70 to 86% protection according to different studies; Monath et al. [18] and Marchetti et al. [15] have observed a higher level of protection when the recombinant sub-unit UreB is complexed with the non-protective sub-unit UreA to form a structure which approaches the conformation of native urease;

(2) the HspA protein, the GroES homologue of *H. pylori*, fused to the maltose binding protein [17];

(3) finally, the native protein of the *H. pylori* cytotoxin (VacA) and its recombinant non-active form are capable of protecting mice against an infectious challenge by a cytotoxin-producing strain (*i.e.* 50% of the strains isolated in clinical assays).

The clearance of a pre-existing infection after active immunization with bacterial sub-units such as those described above also was reported. Corthésy-Theulaz et al. [19] showed clearance after sub-unit UreB, and Ghiara et al. [10] showed immunization with active cytotoxin. These data provide new perspectives for the possible development of immunotherapy for the treatment of *H. pylori* infections.

Prospects for human vaccination

It is now possible to claim that vaccination against *Helicobacter pylori* infections is no longer within the realm of fiction, but is feasible. The mouse, ferret, cat models have proven that immuno-protection can be induced by the administration of recombinant antigens. We must, nevertheless:

(1) demonstrate that the protective efficacy observed in these animal models can also be achieved in a primate model. The physiological differences between the stomachs of these animals and that of humans (differences in acidity and motility) are a limitation that vaccine strategies must circumvent;

(2) define the optimal vaccine formulation, which implies the use of an adjuvant that stimulates mucosal immunity but which is non-toxic for humans. The results of protection studies using the addition of native or detoxified *E. coli* LT toxin (heat-labile enterotoxin) instead of cholera toxin in immunization protocols have already been presented and have proven to be effective, at least in the mouse model. It is obvious that other molecular adjuvants and other means of presentation of identified protective antigens must be studied within the next few years;

(3) it remains vital to understand the basis of the immune response induced during active immunization and to compare it to the response induced in the course of a natural infection.

Such studies will permit evaluation of the possibilities for large scale application to naive pediatric populations for protection and to infected adult populations for treatment.

References

1. Labigne A, Cussac V, Courcoux P. Shuttle cloning and nucleotide sequences of *Helicobacter pylori* genes responsible for urease activity. *J Bacteriol* 1991; 173: 1920-31.
2. Cussac V, Ferrero RL, Labigne A. Expression of *Helicobacter pylori* urease genes in *Escherichia coli* grown under nitrogen-limiting conditions. *J Bacteriol* 1992; 174: 2466-73.
3. Ferrero RL, Labigne A. Cloning, expression and sequencing of *Helicobacter felis* urease genes. *Mol Microbiol* 1993; 9: 323-33.
4. Ferrero RL, Cussac V, Courcoux P, Labigne A. Construction of isogenic urease-negative mutants of *Helicobacter pylori* by allelic exchange. *J Bacteriol* 1992; 174: 4212-7.
5. Eaton K, Krakowka S. Effect of gastric pH on urease-dependent colonization of gnotobiotic piglets by *Helicobacter pylori*. *Infect Immun* 1994; 62: 3604-7.
6. Suerbaum S, Thiberge JM, Kansau I, Ferrero R, Labigne A. *Helicobacter pylori* hspA-B heat shock gene cluster: nucleotide sequence, expression, putative function and immunogenicity. *Mol Microbiol* 1994; 14: 959-74.
7. Chen M, Lee A, Hazell SL, Hu P, Li Y. Immunization against gastric infection with *Helicobacter* species: first step in the prophylaxis of gastric cancer. *Zentralblatt für Bkteriologie* 1993; 280: 155-65.
8. Czinn S, Cai A, Nedrud J. Protection of germ-free mice from infection by *Helicobacter felis* after active oral or passive IgA immunization. *Vaccine* 1993; 11: 637-42.
9. Buck F, Doidge C, Lee A, Hazell S, Manne U, Gust I. Effective protection against *Helicobacter felis* infection in mice with *H. pylori* antigens (abstract). *Am J Gastroenterol* 1994 ; 89: 1335.
10. Ghiara P, Marchetti M, Di Tommaso A, Saletti G, Burroni D, Figura N, Manetti R, Massari P, Marchini A, Arico B, Censini S, Xiang Z, Olivieri R, Pizza MG, De Magistris MT, Abrignani S, Covacci A, Telford JL, Rappuoli R. Infection by *Helicobacter pylori* in a mouse model that mimics human disease: protection by oral vaccination (abstract). *Gut* 1995; 37: 204.
11. Kleanthous H, Tibbits T, Bakos TJ, Goegokopoulos K, Myers G, Ermak TH, *et al. In vivo* selection of a highly adapted *H. pylori* isolate and the development of an *H. pylori* mouse model for studying vaccine efficacy and attenuating lesions. *Gut* 1995; 37 (suppl. 1): A94.

12. Michetti P, Corthésy-Theulaz I, Davin C, Haas R, Vaney AC, Heitz M, Bille J, Kraehenbuhl JP, Saraga E, Blum A. Immunization of BALB/c mice against *Helicobacter felis* infection with *Helicobacter pylori* urease. *Gastroenterology* 1994; 107: 1002-11.
13. Ferrero R, Thiberge JM, Huerre M, Labigne A. Recombinant antigens prepared from the urease subunits of *Helicobacter* spp: evidence of protection in a mouse model of gastric infection. *Infect Immun* 1994; 62: 4981-9.
14. Pappo J, Thomas WD, Kabok Z, Taylor NS, Murphy JC, Fox. Effect of oral immunization with recombinant urease on murine *Helicobacter felis* gastritis. *Infect Immun* 1995; 63: 1246-52.
15. Marchetti M, Arico B, Burroni D, Figura N, Rappuoli R, Ghiara P. Development of a mouse model of *Helicobacter pylori* infection that mimics human disease. *Science* 1995; 267: 1655-8.
16. Cuenca R, Blanchard T, Lee C, Monath T, Redline R, Nedrud J, Czinn S. Therapeutic immunization against *Helicobacter mustelae* infection in naturally infected ferrets. *Gastroenterology* 1995; 108: A78.
17. Ferrero RL, Thiberge JM, Kansau I, Wuscher N, Huerre M, Labigne A. The GroES homolog of *Helicobacter pylori* confers protective immunity against mucosal infection in mice. *Proc Natl Acad Sci USA* 1995; 92: 6499-503.
18. Monath TP, Kleanthous H, Lee CK, Pappo H, Ermak TH, Weltzin R, Ackerman SK. Development of recombinant *Helicobacter pylori* urease as an oral vaccine: current status (abstract). *Gut* 1995; 37: 205.
19. Corthésy-Theulaz I, Vaney AC, Haas R, Saraga E, Kraehenbühl JP, Blum AL, Michetti P. *H. pylori* urease B subunit as a therapeutic vaccine against *H. felis* infection (abstract). *Gastroenterology* 1994; 106: A668.

Recent advances
in gastrointestinal oncology

Helicobacter pylori, gastric cancer and gastric lymphoma

S.G.M. Meuwissen, E.J. Kuipers

Department of Gastroenterology, University Hospital of the « Vrije Universiteit », Amsterdam, The Netherlands

Summary

From several recent epidemiological studies and the WHO report (1994) on this topic, it has become very clear that H. pylori *is responsible for the large majority of gastric cancers. The acquisition of* H. pylori *in childhood is associated with progressive atrophy of the gastric mucosa and most countries with a poor socio-economic status have an increased incidence of gastric cancer. The longer the process of chronic gastritis continues, the larger the chance that mucosal atrophy and dysplasia may indeed occur, as precursor of gastric carcinoma. Alternatively, the incidence of gastric cancer in countries with improvement of their social and economic infrastructure is declining, partly to be attributed to a decline in infection rates of* H. pylori. *Several factors are important in the mechanism of development of gastric cancer, such as dietary factors, smoking, genetic factors of the host, different aggressivity of* H. pylori *strains (heterogeneity, e.g. cagA). The presence of nitrosocompounds and free radicals is important; increased cellular proliferation and epithelial turnover as well as apoptosis may all lead to final mutation. While life-style improvement (diet, smoking) may be of benefit, eradication of* H. pylori *in selected patients may contribute to halting the process of progressive atrophic gastritis and atrophy.* H. pylori *has also been associated with gastric lymphoma, although the mechanisms have not been clarified yet. Eradication of* H. pylori *in low-grade gastric lymphoma has led to impressive improvement, however long-term results are not yet available.*

Helicobacter pylori and gastric cancer

Introduction and epidemiology

A recent Postgraduate Course organised by the EAGE (Nantes, June 1995) has discussed the relationship of *H. pylori* and gastric adenocarcinomas, in particular the epidemiological and histological aspects [1]. This course will deal more in detail with mechanisms of carcinogenesis, natural history of chronic gastritis and the effect of strong acid therapy on the gastric mucosa in *H. pylori* positive patients.

During the last few months many additional reviews have been published, increasing our knowledge on the role of *H. pylori* and gastric cancer. Gastric cancer has declined during recent years, particularly in the developing countries, and it is most likely that improvement of the socioeconomic status in general is one of the major explanatory factors [2, 3]. Many studies have shown that *H. pylori* is responsible for the majority of gastric cancers [4, 5]. One of the most important reviews on the relationship between gastric cancer and *H. pylori* has been published in 1994, discussing all epidemiological aspects involved; this monography from the WHO should be considered as one of the most important reviews up to now [6]. The recognition of *H. pylori* as being responsible for the development of gastric cancer was in particular based on the overall analysis of several clinical studies relating higher prevalences of *H. pylori* with higher incidences of gastric cancer in different countries and on prospective cohort studies showing an increased cancer risk in infected subjects. A recent review has analysed all epidemiological arguments in favour of a role of *H. pylori* in the development of gastric cancer [7].

The decline in incidence rates of gastric cancer run parallel to those of chronic *H. pylori* gastritis. Studies from Finland have convincingly demonstrated that the age specific prevalence of *H. pylori* gastritis has decreased during recent years, which is most likely due to lower risk of acquiring *H. pylori* during childhood (birth-cohort dependent phenomenon) [8]; a similar observation was recently reported from the Netherlands [9]. These recent data confirm the results from previous studies [10, 11]. The lower prevalence of *H. pylori* chronic gastritis as well as the active eradication of *H. pylori* in many individuals, who have been shown to be *H. pylori* positive, will undoubtedly have effect on the incidence of gastric cancer in the forthcoming years. However this statement will hold true only for those countries with steadily improving environmental hygiene, in which housing conditions are improved, crowding of families is avoided and where water supply of good quality can be guaranteed.

Mechanisms of gastric carcinogenesis *(Figure 1)*

Which factors are important in the development of gastric cancer?

• **Duration of *H. pylori* infection.** *H. pylori* has not been characterised as mutagenic. The process of chronic mucosal inflammation, in which bacterial products as well as host inflammatory products are involved during a long time period may however ultimately lead to atrophy, dysplasia and finally cancer. A significant trend towards an increased odds ratio for the development of gastric cancer was shown with longer intervals between collection of sera and development of cancer in different prospective series and this undoubtedly reflects the extended time period (many years) before this process of chronic inflammation leads to malignancy [12]. A mathematical model has been developed to describe the time relationship between length of *H. pylori* infection and risk of developing gastric cancer; the well-known increased incidence of gastric cancer in black Americans compared with white could be contributed to differences in length of *H. pylori* exposure by race [13].

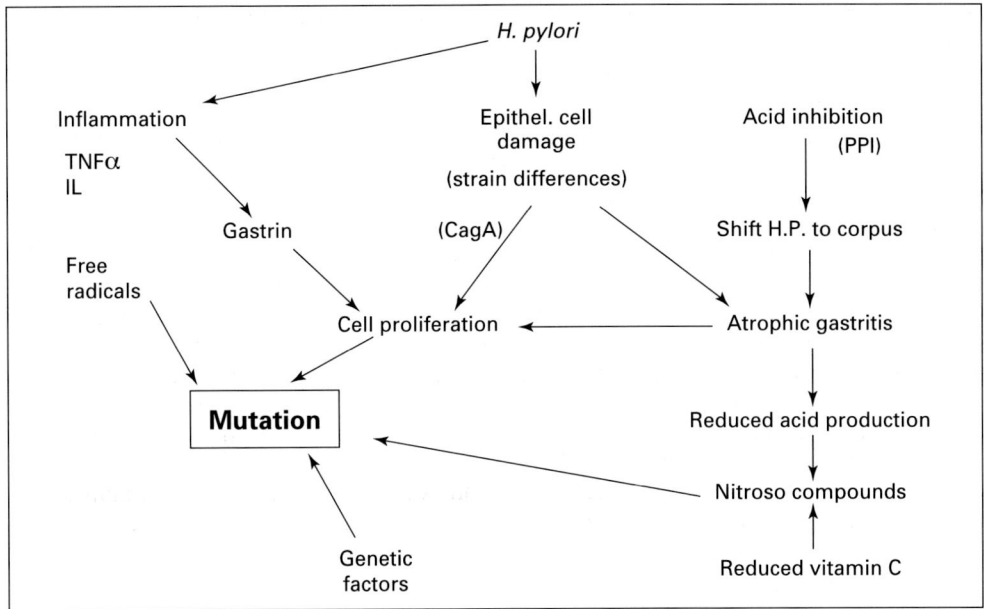

Figure 1. A simplified flow diagram, depicting possible mechanisms involved in the development of gastric cancer (« Mutation »).

- **Heterogeneity of *H. pylori*.** The heterogeneous nature of *H. pylori* has now well been established, 60 % of the different strains possess the cagA gene (cytotoxin-associated gene A), a gene encoding a high molecular weight immunodominant antigen (120-128 kDa) [14, 15]. This gene is part of a 30 kb pathogenicity island on the genome of *H. pylori*, which contains several other genes like picA and picB. All these genes play a role in the pathogenicity of *H. pylori* infections. Phenotypically one may distinct two types: type I: expression of cagA and vacA (vacuolating toxin) and type II: absence of these two proteins [16]. The value of using this phenotypic classification has not been established as yet. Induction of interleukin-8 protein in gastric epithelial cells *(in vitro)* takes in particular place with type I strain *H. pylori* [17, 18]. It has been suggested that cagA not in itself is responsible for cytokine induction, but other gene products from the cagA « region ». Epithelial neutrophilic infiltration has been associated with cagA expression [19] and with raised serum pepsinogen levels as markers of mucosal inflammation [20]. In a long-term follow-up study of Japanese American men in Hawaii, it was demonstrated that cagA + individuals carry an increased risk of developing gastric cancer (O.R.1.9; 95 % CI 0.9-4.0) [21]. The cagA status was found to be associated with an increased risk for the development of atrophic gastritis and intestinal metaplasia in a long-term follow-up study of 11.5 y (O.R. 3.48; 95 % C.I. 1.02-12.18) [22]. An association has been shown with intestinal metaplasia, developing in patients with dyspepsia (O.R. 4.75; 95 % C.I. 1.31-17.9) [23]. In black Americans the risk for developing gastric cancer is increased, possibly related to the total duration of infection. A mathematical model was developed to describe such time relationship; the increased incidence of gastric cancer in black Americans could indeed be contributed to differences in length of *H. pylori* exposure by race [13]; in addition, the proportion of cagA + black individuals was found to be higher than in white

(79.4 % versus 50 %; O.R. 5.0; 95 C.I. 1.6-15.3) [24]. A recent study showed that type I *H. pylori* infection (cagA+) was an independent risk factor for gastric cancer patients with intestinal type gastric cancer, but not the diffuse type gastric cancer (O.R. 3.7; 95 % C.I. 1.7-8.3) [25]. However these data differed from those observed in a German study [26]. The above data taken together strongly suggest that the expression of the cagA protein is associated with an increased risk for developing atrophic gastritis and gastric cancer.

• **Ascorbic acid (vitamin C).** *H. pylori* associated gastritis and therefore the development of gastric cancer is linked to a significant decrease of vitamin C levels in the gastric juice, which cannot be corrected by increased oral intake of vitamin C, until eradication of *H. pylori* has taken place [27-29]. It is most likely that the scavenger function of vitamin C of reactive oxygen products which are present during chronic *H. pylori* infection is reduced until after therapy. Without eradication, no inhibition occurs of N-nitrosation [30].

• **Epithelial turnover and apoptosis.** It has been shown that epithelial turnover is increased in patients with *H. pylori* gastritis, as demonstrated by a significant higher labelling index % (LI %), in comparison to *H. pylori* negative subjects or controls [31], which may lead to hyperproliferation of the gastric epithelium. One of the mechanisms likely to be involved is apoptosis or programmed cell death. A careful balance exists between cell proliferation and cell death, and the regulation of the latter mechanism has only been appreciated recently [32, 33]. Resistance to programmed cell death may occur through overexpression of the oncogene bcl2 or bcl2 family members, such as bclx and this has been shown to occur for gastric cancer [34]. In the *H. pylori* uninfected stomach apoptotic cells are rare and are found mainly superficially, in contrast to the infected stomach; in the latter group the apoptotic rate rose from 2.9 (controls) to 16.8 % of epithelial cells, falling to 3.1 % after therapy [35]. It has been documented that *H. pylori* induces NO synthase expression; recently it was shown in rabbit gastric epithelial cells that *H. pylori* induces apoptosis (NO-mediated apoptosis) [36]. Ammonia may also be involved *via* the formation of monochloramine (NH_2Cl), inducing apoptosis *in vitro* [37]. Cytokines such as IFNγ and TNFα may also be involved in this process, inducing apoptosis [38]. The *H. pylori* mediated apoptosis in the gastric epithelium was not associated with expression of p53 in the same tissue [39]. In conclusion: it is extremely likely, that induction of apoptosis plays a significant role in human *H. pylori* associated gastric carcinogenesis and unravelling the molecular basis of the genes involved and respective induction mechanisms may be of major importance.

Chronic atrophic gastritis as precursor of gastric atrophy and gastric cancer

It has been well established that chronic *H. pylori* gastritis may lead to atrophy and intestinal metaplasia, with an increased risk for gastric cancer. The prevalence of atrophy among adults increases by 1-3 % annually, as shown in several studies, not yet taking into account the presence of *H. pylori* [40-42]; in our recent study, *H. pylori* was shown to be an important risk factor for the development of chronic atrophic gastritis and intestinal metaplasia, the annual increase of atrophic corpus gastritis corresponding with the literature data as shown above (1.15 %, 0.6-1.8 %) (*H. pylori* -: 0.3 % and *H. pylori* +: 1.8 %) [43]. Only recently it has been appreciated that strong gastric acid suppression may profoundly influence the normal acidic habitat of *H. pylori* and influence activity of corpus gastritis, thereby increasing the speed of atrophic changes. Changes in the intragastric distribution of *H. pylori* during treatment with a PPI were observed by Vigneri *et al.*, Logan *et al.* and Marzio *et al.* [44-46] and described in detail by our group [47]. It was shown that, after 8 weeks therapy with a PPI, a predominant inflammatory reaction of the corpus occurred in *H. pylori* + patients, with increase in the corpus of an inflammatory score and decrease of the inflammatory activity in the antrum [47]. Long-term omeprazole therapy given to patients with reflux oesophagitis during a follow-up study of several years produced an increase of the annual rate of development of atrophic gastritis from 0.8 % in *H. pylori* - patients to 6.1 % in the *H. pylori* + group (95 % CI: 3.8-8.8). Argyrophil-cell hyperplasia increased as well in the *H. pylori* + group [48]. Therefore strong arguments are available to suggest that *H. pylori* + patients who are to receive long-term strong acid suppression, should have eradication therapy at the start of their therapy. The mechanisms by which gastric atrophy occurs are poorly understood. One attractive possibility may be that lipopolysaccharides (LPS) of *H. pylori* express Lewis y and x blood group structures; the beta chain of gastric H+,K+ ATP-ase contains Lewis y epitopes. Anti-Lewis y (and x) antibodies may then bind to the proton pump and initiate a process of parietal cell inactivation, gastric inflammation and finally atrophy [49]. Whether such autoimmune mechanism may be responsible for the striking and progressive chronic and progressive atrophic gastritis, remains to be confirmed by prospective studies.

Helicobacter pylori and gastric lymphoma

Helicobacter pylori has been associated to the development of gastric lymphomas (MALT lymphoma) and epidemiological data support the principal pathogenic role of *H. pylori* in the development of gastric lymphoma [50, 51]. *H. pylori* has been detected in 92 % of patients with MALT lymphoma [52], up to 97 % in a German study [53]. An excellent review of all data has been presented at the EAGE (Nantes, June 1995) by Ruskoné-Fourmestraux [54].

MALT (mucosa associated lymphoid tissue) is found abundantly in the gastrointestinal tract, for example in the Peyer's patches, however in the stomach in principle no lymphoid tissue is detected except in children and young adults [55]. The presence of MALT in the stomach is indicative for *H. pylori* infection: chronic *H. pylori* infection is associated with B-cell hyperplasia, B-cell follicles with germinal centres within the gastric mucosa, in addition to plasmacytosis [56]. MALT lymphomas are characterised by a monoclonal B cell population, infiltrating the epithelium (« lymphoepithelial lesions ») by small cleaved or centrocyte-like cells, with a smaller percentage of larger blasts also being present [57, 58]. The lymphoid follicles are thought to be present due the chronic antigenic stimulation of *H. pylori*, the lymphoproliferative process finally becoming autonomous, developing a neoplastic character [54, 56]. After *H. pylori* eradication, the density of the lymphoplasmacellular infiltrate decreases considerably. The exact mechanisms how *H. pylori* triggers the development of MALT lymphoma remain unknown. The classic *in vitro* study by Hussell has shown that low-grade primary B-cell gastric MALT lymphoma cells show a proliferative response to *H. pylori* only in the presence of non-neoplastic T lymphocytes, while removal of these cells from the culture abolished this response; this T cell dependency is likely to be of major importance [59]. The relation of *H. pylori* and B-cell clonality was recently studied in patients with dyspepsia; surprisingly VDJ clonality was observed equally frequent in patients with and without the presence of *H. pylori* detectable, suggesting that other factors (genetic, immunological) may also be important [60]. Genetic factors are most likely to play a role, allelic imbalance was shown to be present in 5 of 12 patients with MALT lymphoma (at the DCC locus or APC locus) [61]. Other factors, such as intercurrent infections, dietary factors or unknown disorders of the immune system, may also be important.

Regression of low-grade MALT lymphoma after therapy

Regression has been observed by an increasing number of authors, after the initial publication by Wotherspoon *et al.* [62]. This study described in 5 of 6 patients with a low-grade MALT lymphoma, in whom *H. pylori* was eradicated, disappearance of the MALT lymphoma during the time of observation (4-10 months). In 1994, a case report on the disappearance of a large low-grade MALT lymphoma in the stomach was described after adequate anti-*H. pylori* therapy [63]. The largest series has been published recently at the AGA-meeting (San Francisco) as an abstract by a German group: 37 of 50 (74 %) patients with a low-grade B-cell lymphoma showed complete histological regression of the tumor after *H. pylori* eradication (median follow-up 5 months), 5 cases showed partial regression (10 %) and 6 cases needed either surgery or chemotherapy (16 %) [64]. In most patients in whom regression was documented, no recurrences had occurred after 24 months. An important study from Italy in 68 patients with low-grade MALT lymphoma of the stomach, who were eradicated, showed during a follow-up of 6-36 months histologic regression in 90 %, however disappearance of monoclonality occurred in 45 % only [65]. Smaller series with good results have been reported as well [66, 67]. One should however keep in mind that diagnostic means to evaluate potential recurrences have been different in the above studies. Several studies have shown that endoscopic ultrasonography should be used for the evaluation of recurrent disease after therapy, in order to avoid false negative biopsy results [68, 69].

In conclusion, *H. pylori* eradication in patients with low-grade MALT lymphoma is of major importance and should be advocated strongly. In contrast, in high-grade MALT lymphoma patients, antibacterial therapy is not primary therapy of choice, but may be of some additional value [70].

References

1. Sipponen P. *H. pylori* and adenocarcinomas. Postgraduate course UEDW, Nantes 1995.
2. Howson C, Hiyama T, Wynder E. The decline in gastric cancer epidemiology of an unplanned triumph. *Epidemiol Rev* 1986; 8: 1-27.
3. Coleman MP, Esteve J, Damieck P, et al. *Trends in cancer incidence and mortality.* Lyon: IARC Scientific Publications, 1993.
4. Talley NJ, Zinsmeister AR, Weaver A, et al. Gastric adenocarcinoma and *Helicobacter pylori* infection. *J Natl Cancer Inst* 1991; 83: 1734-9.
5. Craanen M, Blok P, Dekker W, Tytgat G. *H. pylori* and early gastric cancer. *Gut* 1994; 35: 1372-4.
6. International Agency for Research on Cancer. IARC Monographs on the evaluation of carcinogenic risks to humans, Vol 61, *Schistosomes, liver flukes and Helicobacter pylori.* Lyon, 1994.

7. Webb P, Forman D. *Helicobacter pylori* as a risk factor for cancer. *Clin Gastroenterol* 1995; 9: 563-82.
8. Sipponen P, Kekki M, Seppala K, Siurala M. The relationships between chronic gastritis and gastric acid secretion. *Aliment Pharmacol Ther* 1996; 10 (suppl 1): 103-18.
9. Roosendaal R, Kuipers E, Meuwissen S, Vandenbroucke-Grauls C. *Helicobacter pylori* and the birth-cohort effect: evidence for continuous decrease of infection rates in childhood. *Gastroenterology* 1996; 110: A242.
10. Parsonnet J, Blaser MJ, Pérez-Pérez GI, et al. Symptoms and risk factors of *Helicobacter pylori* in a cohort of epidemiologists. *Gastroenterology* 1992; 102: 41-6.
11. Banatvala N, Mayo K, Mégraud F, Jennings R, Deeks JJ, Feldman RA. The cohort effect and *Helicobacter pylori*. *J Infect Dis* 1993; 168: 219-21.
12. Forman D, Webb P, Parsonnet J. *Helicobacter pylori* and gastric cancer. *Lancet* 1994; 343: 243-4.
13. Kim W, Therneau T, Locke G, Dickson E. Quantifying the role of *H. pylori* in gastric carcinogenesis: an accelerated failure time model. *Gastroenterology* 1996; 110: A156.
14. Taylor DE, Eaton M, Chang N, Salama SM. Construction of a *Helicobacter pylori* genome map and demonstration of diversity at the genome level. *J Bacteriol* 1992; 174: 6800-6.
15. Covacci A, Censini S, Bugnoli M, et al. Molecular characterization of the 128-kDa immunodominant antigen of *Helicobacter pylori* associated with cytotoxicity and duodenal ulcer. *Proc Natl Acad Sci USA* 1993; 90: 5791-5.
16. Xiang Z, Censini S, Bayeli P, Telford J, Figura N, Rappuoli R. Analysis of expression of CagA and VacA virulence factors in 43 strains of *Helicobacter pylori* reveals that clinical isolates can be divided into two major types and that CagA is not necessary fot expression of the vacuolating cytotoxin. *Infect Immun* 1995; 63: 94-8.
17. Crabtree J, Farmery S, Lindley I, Figura N, Peichl P, Tompkins D. CagA/cytotoxic strains of *Helicobacter pylori* and interleukin-8 expression in gastric epithelial cells. *J Clin Pathol* 1994; 47: 945-50.
18. Crabtree J, Covacci A, Farmery S, Ziang Z, Tompkins D. *Helicobacter pylori* induced interleukin-8 expression in gastric epithelial cells is associated with CagA positive phenotype. *J Clin Pathol* 1995; 48: 41-5.
19. Crabtree JE, Taylor JD, Wyatt JI, et al. Mucosal IgA recognition of *Helicobacter pylori* 120 kDa protein, peptic ulceration, and gastric pathology. *Lancet* 1991; 338: 332-5.
20. Oderda G, Figura N, Bayeli PF, et al. Serologic IgG recognition of *Helicobacter pylori* cytotoxin-associated protein, peptic ulcer and gastroduodenal pathology in childhood. *Eur J Gastroenterol Hepatol* 1993; 5: 695-9.
21. Blaser MJ, Pérez-Pérez GI, Kleanthous H, et al. Infection with *Helicobacter pylori* strains possessing *cagA* is associated with an increased risk of developing adenocarcinoma of the stomach. *Cancer Res* 1995; 55: 2111-5.
22. Kuipers E, Perez-Perez G, Meuwissen S, Blaser M. *Helicobacter pylori* and atrophic gastritis: importance of the CagA status. *J Natl Canc Inst* 1995; 87 (23): 1777-80.
23. Crabtree J, Wyatt J, Perry S, Davies G, Covacci A, Morgan A. CagA seropositive *Helicobacter pylori* infected non-ulcer patients have increased frequency of intestinal metaplasia. *Gastroenterology* 1996; 110 (4): A85.
24. Parsonnet J, Replogle M, Yang S, Hiatt R. Prevalence of the type I *H. pylori* phenotype differs among ethnic/racial groups in the San Francisco bay area. *Gastroenterology* 1996; 110: A221.
25. Parsonnet J, Friedman G, Orentreich N, Vogelman J. Infection with the type I phenotype of *H. pylori* increases risk for gastric cancer independent of corpus atrophy. *Gastroenterology* 1996; 110: A221.
26. Rudi J, Kolb C, Maiwald M, Zuna I, Galle P, Stremmel W. Serum antibodies against the *Helicobacter pylori* proteins Cag-A and Vac-A are associated with an increased risk for gastric carcinoma. *Gastroenterology* 1996; 110: A245.
27. Sobala GM, Schorah CJ, Sanderson M, et al. Ascorbic acid in the human stomach. *Gastroenterology* 1989; 97: 357-63.

28. Sobala G, Schorah C, Shires S, et al. Effect of eradication of *Helicobacter pylori* on gastric juice ascorbic acid concentrations. *Gut* 1993; 34: 1038-41.
29. Rood J, Ruiz B. *Helicobacter pylori*-associated gastritis and the ascorbic acid concentration in gastric juice. *Nutr Cancer* 1994; 22: 65-72.
30. Mirvish S. Experimental evidence for inhibition of N-nitroso compound formation as a factor in the negative correlation between Vitamin C consumption and the incidence of certain cancers. *Cancer Res* 1994; 54 (suppl.): 1948s-1951s.
31. Cahill R, Sant S, Beattie S, Hamilton H, O'Morain C. *Helicobacter pylori* and increased epithelial cell proliferation: a risk factor for cancer. *Eur J Gastroenterol Hepatol* 1994; 94: 1123-7.
32. Thompson C. Apoptosis in the pathogenesis and treatment of disease. *Science* 1995; 267: 1456-60.
33. Hall P, Coates P, Ansari B, Hopwood D. Regulation of cell number in the mammalian gastrointestinal tract: the importance of apoptosis. *J Cell Sci* 1994; 107: 3569-77.
34. Lauwers G, Scott G, Hendricks J. Immunohistochemical evidence of aberrant bcl-2 protein expression in gastric epithelial dysplasia. *Cancer* 1994; 73: 2900-4.
35. Moss S, Calam J, Agarwal B, Wang S, Holt P. Induction of gastric epithelial apoptosis by *Helicobacter pylori*. *Gut* 1996; 38: 498-501.
36. Fukuda T, Arakawa T, Fujiwara Y, Nakagawa K, Uno H. Nitric oxide induces apoptosis in gastric mucosal cells *in vitro*. *Gastroenterology* 1996; 110: A111.
37. Naito Y, Yoshikawa T, Yagi N, Boku Y, Vemura M. Cell growth inhibition and apoptosis induced by monochloramine in a gastric mucosal cell line. *Gastroenterology* 1996; 110: A205.
38. Behar S, vanHouten N, Bamford K, Reyes V, Crowe S, Ernst P. *H. pylori* induces apoptosis in gastric epithelial cells which is enhanced by cytokines from TH1 cells. *Gastroenterology* 1996; 110: A862.
39. Jones N, Yeger H, Cutz E, Sherman P. *Helicobacter pylori* induces apoptosis of gastric antral epithelial cells *in vivo*. *Gastroenterology* 1996; 110: A933.
40. Sipponen P. Long-term consequences of gastroduodenal inflammation. *Eur J Gastroenterol Hepatol* 1992; 4 (suppl 2): S25-9.
41. Correa P, Haenszel W, Cuello C, et al. Gastric precancerous process in a high risk population: cross-sectional studies. *Cancer Res* 1990; 50: 4731-6.
42. Villako K, Kekki M, Maaroos HI, et al. Chronic gastritis: progression of inflammation and atrophy in a six-year endoscopic follow-up of a random sample of 142 Estonian urban subjects. *Scand J Gastroenterol* 1991; 26 (suppl. 186): 135-41.
43. Kuipers EJ, Uyterlinde AM, Peña AS, et al. Long term sequelae of *Helicobacter pylori* gastritis. *Lancet* 1995; 345: 1525-8.
44. Vigneri S, Termini R, Scialabba A, et al. Omeprazole long-term treatment for duodenal ulcer: effects on the gastric distribution of *Helicobacter pylori*. *Acta Gastroenterol Belg* 1993; 56 (suppl.): 147.
45. Logan RPH, Walker MM, Misiewicz JJ, Gummett PA, Karim QN, Baron JH. Changes in the intragastric distribution of *Helicobacter pylori* during treatment with omeprazole. *Gut* 1995; 36: 12-6.
46. Marzio L, Biasco G, Cifani F, deFanis C, Falcucci M, Ferrini G. Short-and long-term omeprazole for the treatment and prevention of duodenal ulcer, and effect on *Helicobacter pylori*. *Am J Gastroenterol* 1995; 90: 2172-6.
47. Kuipers EJ, Uyterlinde AM, Peña AS, et al. Increase of *Helicobacter pylori* associated corpus gastritis during acid suppressive therapy. Implications for long-term safety. *Am J Gastroenterol* 1995; 90: 1401-6.
48. Kuipers E, Lundell L, Klinkenberg-Knol E, Havu N, Festen H. Atrophic gastritis and *Helicobacter pylori* in patients with reflux esophagitis treated with omeprazole or fundoplication. *N Engl J Med* 1996; 334: 1018-22.
49. Appelmelk J, Simoons-Smit I, Negrini R, et al. Potential role of molecular mimicry between *Helicobacter pylori* lipopolysaccharide and host lewis blood group antigens in autoimmunity. *Infect Immun* 1996; 64: 2031-40.

50. Doglioni C, Wotherspoon A, Maschini A, deBoni M, Isaacson P. High incidence of primary gastric lymphoma in Northeastern Italy. *Lancet* 1992; 339: 834-5.
51. Genta R, Segura A, Gutierrez O, Velasco B, Graham D, Shahab I. High incidence of unsuspected gastric lymphoma of the mucosa associated lymphoid tissue in a population at high risk for gastric cancer. *Gastroenterology* 1996; 110: A517.
52. Wotherspoon A, Ortiz-Hidalgo C, Falzon M, Isaacson P. *Helicobacter pylori*-associated gastritis and primary B-cell gastric lymphoma. *Lancet* 1991; 338: 1175-6.
53. Eidt S, Stolte M, Fischer R. *Helicobacter pylori* gastritis and primary gastric non-Hodgkin's lymphomas. *J Clin Pathol* 1994; 47: 436-9.
54. Ruskoné-Fourmestraux A. *Helicobacter pylori* and gastric lymphoma. EAGE 1995; Nantes.
55. McCormick C, Symmans P, Levison D. Mucosa associated lymphoid tissue. *GI Cancer* 1995; 1: 9-13.
56. Genta RM, Hamner HW, Graham DY. Gastric lymphoid follicles in *Helicobacter pylori* infection. *Hum Pathol* 1993; 24: 577-83.
57. Parsonnet J, Hansen S, Rodriguez L, *et al. Helicobacter pylori* infection and gastric lymphoma. *N Engl J Med* 1994; 330: 1267-71.
58. Ruskoné-Fourmestraux A, Aegerter P, Delmer A, *et al.* Primary digestive tract lymphoma: a prospective multicentric study of 91 patients. *Gastroenterology* 1993; 105: 1662-71.
59. Hussell T, Isaacson P, Crabtree J, Spencer J. The response of cells from low-grade B-cell gastric lymphomas of mucosa-associated lymphoid tissue to *Helicobacter pylori. Lancet* 1993; 342: 571-4.
60. Sorrentino D, Ferraccioli G, deVita S, *et al.* B-cell clonality and infection with *Helicobacter pylori*: implications for development of gastric lymphoma. *Gut* 1996; 38: 837-40.
61. Calvert R, Randerson J, Evans P, *et al.* Genetic abnormalities during transition from *Helicobacter pylori*-associated gastritis to low-grade MALToma. *Lancet* 1995; 345: 26-7.
62. Wotherspoon A, Doglioni C, Diss T, *et al.* Regression of primary low-grade B-cell gastric lymphoma of mucosa-associated lymphoid tissue type after eradication of *Helicobacter pylori. Lancet* 1993; 342: 575-7.
63. Weber D, Dimopoulos M, Anandu D, Pugh W, Steinbach G. Regression of gastric lymphoma of mucosa-associated lymphoid tissue with antibiotic therapy for *Helicobacter pylori. Gastroenterology* 1994; 107: 1835-8.
64. Bayerdorffer E, Morgner A, Neubauer A, *et al.* Regression of primary gastric MALT lymphoma after cure of *Helicobacter pylori* infection: a two-year follow-up report of the German MALT lymphoma trial. *Gastroenterology* 1996; 110: A490.
65. Franzin G, Zamboni G, Savio A, *et al.* Gastric MALT low-grade lymphoma: follow-up study after eradication of *Helicobacter pylori. Gastroenterology* 1996; 110: A109.
66. Boot H, Jong Dd, Heerde PV, Burgers J, Taal B. Role of *Helicobacter pylori* eradication in low grade and high grade gastric malt lymphoma-early results. *Gastroenterology* 1996; 110: A493.
67. Fischbach W, Kolve M, Engemann R, Greiner A, Stolte M. Unexpected success of *Helicobacter pylori* eradication in low grade MALT lymphoma. *Gastroenterology* 1996: A512.
68. Sackmann M, Morgner A, Rudolph R, *et al.* Regression of MALT lymphoma following eradication of *Helicobacter pylori* is predicted by endosonographic staging. *Gastroenterology* 1996; 110: A586.
69. Levy M, Hammel P, Lamarque D, *et al.* Endoscopic ultrasonography (EUS) for initial staging and follow-up in MALT gastric lymphoma (MGL) medically treated. *Gastroenterology* 1996; 110: A551.
70. Boot H, Jong Dd, Heerde Pv, Taal B. Role of *Helicobacter pylori* eradication in high-grade MALT-lymphoma. *Lancet* 1995: 346.

Octreoscan scintigraphy in endocrine gastroenteropancreatic tumors

G. Cadiot[1], R. Lebtahi[2], D. Le Guludec[2], M. Mignon[1]

[1] Service d'Hépato-Gastroentérologie, [2] Service de Médecine Nucléaire, CHU Bichat-Claude Bernard, Paris, France

Summary

Most endocrine gastroenteropancreatic (GEP) tumors, except insulinomas, carry a high density of somatostatin receptors that allow their detection in vivo using an indium-labelled octreotide (Octreoscan scintigraphy). Octreoscan scintigraphy adds useful complementary information to other imaging techniques, including endoscopic ultrasonography. Its major benefit is the detection of previously unknown metastatic or primary tumors in 10 to 50 % of the patients. The sensitivity varies with the location and the size of the tumors, which is very high for liver metastases (> 90 %). Despite the presence of somatostatin receptors in other types of tumors or pathological tissues, the Octreoscan specificity is very high (> 95 %) in patients with known endocrine tumors. First results suggest that the impact of Octreoscan scintigraphy on patient management is very high, with modifications in management in 25 % to 50 % of patients. This is still currently under evaluation in other series. The main established indications for Octreoscan scintigraphy are the preoperative evaluation of the tumoral spread and the differenciation with other lesions evidenced by other imaging modalities.

Endocrine gastroenteropancreatic (GEP) tumors are often small, sometimes multiple and may metastasize in lymph nodes, liver, bones and chest. Since surgery is the only in cure, precise preoperative localization of all the tumors (primary and metastases) is fundamental. Unfortunately, conventional and even more recent imaging techniques such as endoscopic ultrasonography, often do not visualize all the tumors.

The possibility to detect tumors bearing somatostatin receptors (SSTR) using Octreoscan scintigraphy (^{111}-In-Pentetreotide) has been a considerable advancement in this field [1-2]. This review reports on the current knowledge of the usefulness of Octreoscan scintigraphy in patients with endocrine GEP tumors, with special reference to recent data and our experience.

Somatostatin receptors

Five subtypes of human SSTR have been cloned [3-6]. Octreotide, the labelled somatostatin analogue used for Octreoscan scintigraphy, binds with high affinity to SSTR2, and with low affinity to the other subtypes [6-7].

Most endocrine tumors contain one or several subtypes of SSTR. More than 80 % of endocrine GEP tumors, except insulinomas, contain octreotide receptors or SSTR2 and may theorically be visualized with Octreoscan scintigraphy [2, 8] *(Table I)*. Fewer insulinomas contain SSTR2 *(Table I)*. Well differentiated tumors might express SSTR more often than undifferentiated tumors [10].

Table I. Number and percentage of endocrine gastroenteropancreatic tumors bearing octreotide receptors or SSTR2 *in vitro* (modified from [2, 7-9])

Tumor type	Nb positive tumors	(% positive tumors)
Duodenopancreatic tumors		
Gastrinomas	13/13	(100)
Unclassified	4/4	(100)
Insulinomas	18/27	(67)
Glucagonomas	2/2	(100)
Carcinoids	55/62	(88)

Non-endocrine tumors such as in breast cancer, lymphomas, nervous system tumors or pathological non-tumoral tissues such as granulomatous diseases and chronic inflammation often contain a high density of SSTR2 (for review, see [2]). In clinical practice, however the fact that tissues other than endocrine tumors may be visualized by Octreoscan scintigraphy, except for postoperative inflammation, is not a limiting factor in a patient with endocrine tumors.

Autoradiographic *in vitro* studies have shown that exocrine pancreatic tumors do not express SSTR [11]. This strongly suggests that pancreatic tumors visualized by Octreoscan scintigraphy are not adenocarcinomas.

Technical considerations

The tracer used is [^{111}-In-DTPA-D-Phe ^{1}]-octreotide (*i.e.*, ^{111}-In-Pentetreotide) (Mallinckrodt diagnostica) [12]. The half-life time is 2.8 days allowing late images (up to 48 hr) to be performed. Most of the tracer is cleared *via* the kidneys. The digestive clearance of the tracer after hepatobiliary secretion may create abdominal artefacts. Laxatives must be administered prior to and during the examination. We use PEG 4000 [9, 13]. Physiological accumulation of the tracer is noted in the liver, the spleen, the kidneys, the urinary bladder, the pituitary, the thyroid, the salivary glands and sometimes the galbladder.

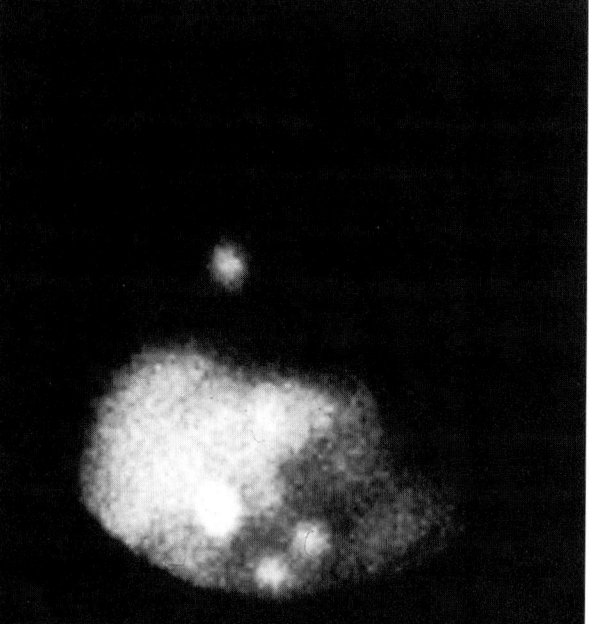

Figure 2. Octreoscan scintigraphy (anterior view of the upper abdomen and the chest) in a patient with the Zollinger-Ellison syndrome and multiple endocrine neoplasia type 1: chest hot spot corresponding to a previously unknown mediastinal metastatic lymph node; heterogeneity of the left lobe of the liver corresponding to previously unknown metastases; hot spots in the duodenopancreatic area corresponding to a duodenal gastrinoma and metastatic lymph nodes.

Detection of gastroenteropancreatic tumors with Octreoscan scintigraphy

Octreoscan scintigraphy may visualize previously known primary and secondary tumors, when they contain SSTR2. Its major advantage is to discover previously unknown primary or metastatic tumors in 10 to 54 % of the patients, according to different series, in areas that are hardly explored by conventional imaging techniques [1-2, 8, 13, 16-29]. In patients with MEN1, endocrine tumors other than abdominal ones might also be discovered, especially thymic or bronchial carcinoids [13, 23]. Octreoscan scintigraphy is helpful in the diagnosis of late postoperative recurrence (when the resected tumors are Octreoscan-positive) or in the interpretation of a doubtful image with conventional imaging. According to some authors, results of Octreoscan scintigraphy are helpful for initiating somatostatin analog therapy [2, 19, 20, 22, 30, 31].

Global positive rates in gastroenteropancreatic tumors

The global positive rates of Octreoscan scintigraphy for most endocrine tumors, except insulinomas, has been set at 70-100 % according to different experiences *(Tables II to IV)*. These percentages highly parallel the percentages of tumors expressing SSTR *(Table I)*. In the 2 largest series of patients with the Zollinger-Ellison syndrome (ZES) studied in a single institution, the global positive rates were 69 % [23] and 70 % [24] *(Table III)*. It is much probable that most metastases derived from a primary tumor visualized with whereas 47 % (8/17) of the tumors visualized by Octreoscan scintigraphy measured less than 15 mm (P = 0. 017) [9]. A German study also showed that only 35 % of pancreatic tumors measuring less than 2 cm were detected as compared to 87 % of tumors measuring more than 2 cm [17]. However, this series included small insulinomas which might be SSTR-negative.

Sensitivity probably also depends on the tumor location. In a large series, gastrinomas located in the duodenopancreatic area (sensitivity 58 to 70 %) are more difficult to visualize than hepatic gastrinomas (90-100 %) [13, 23-24, 26, 32-34]; the detection rate of duodenal gastrinomas is low, 38 % to 46 % [9, 25]. A higher detection rate for liver metastases than for primary tumors (pancreas, intestine) has also been observed in patients with different types of endocrine tumors [18, 22]. The fact that primary tumors are often smaller and less numerous than liver metastases might also explain such a difference. However, a high background of radioactivity seems to be a limiting factor in the duodenopancreatic area.

Tumors located close to each other, for example a duodenal gastrinoma and a tumoral lymph node, might be difficult to separate from each other, since hot spots might merge [9, 13]. Tumors might also be hidden by an organ visualized physiologically with Octreoscan scintigraphy (liver, kidney, spleen) [13]. This emphasizes the need for systematically performing SPET and/or multiple lateral and oblique planar views.

Improvement of tumoral detection with Octreoscan scintigraphy

Despite these limiting factors, Octreoscan scintigraphy dramatically improves the detection of endocrine GEP tumors, whatever their localization, since conventional imaging techniques are not sensitive enough to detect small GEP tumors [9, 13, 24, 35-36]. For example, Octreoscan scintigraphy was in our hands the only positive imaging technique in 32 % of the patients with duodenal and lymph nodes gastrinomas [9]. Performing both endoscopic ultrasonography and Octreoscan scintigraphy, in which both have individually a rate of 58 % positivity, increased the detection rate of gastrinomas to 90 % [9]. This is a feature that has only been noted with very invasive techniques such as angiography with venous gastrin measurement after secretin stimulation [35]. In patients with digestive carcinoid tumors, Octreoscan is often the only technique able to detect the primary site in the intestine. In this indication the sensitivity of Octreoscan scintigraphy is 66-100 % [22].

Octreoscan scintigraphy is very useful in the case of doubtful images with conventional imaging techniques in a patient with known endocrine tumors. Octreoscan scintigraphy distinguishes bone metastases from other bone pathologies and is more sensitive and much more specific than conventional bone scintigraphy [37, 38]. In a series of ZES patients with hepatic lesions that could not be differentiated between hemangiomas or metastases, Octreoscan scintigraphy was positive in 95 % of cases with metastases and 0 % of cases of hepatic hemangiomas, with positive and negative predictive values for metastases of 100 % and 94 %, respectively [34].

Specificity is high when artefactual images due to the digestive accumulation of the tracer (easy to discard when scintigraphic images are redone a few hours after) or to focal inflammation (easy to discard clinically) are excluded [2]. In the context of a patient with proven endocrine tumor, specificity is at least 90 %, reaching 100 % in several series [19, 22, 26, 33, 39]. Due to its cost and to the fact that other types of tumoral and nontumoral pathologies can be visualized by Octreoscan scintigraphy, we think that Octreoscan scintigraphy should not be used to ascertain a diagnosis of endocrine tumor in a patient with atypical symptoms (for example, unexplained diarrhoea). However, Octreoscan scintigraphy should be performed in a patient with an asymptomatic pancreatic tumor which is most likely to be endocrine when Octreoscan scintigraphy is positive [11].

Clinical relevance of Octreoscan scintigraphy

That Octreoscan scintigraphy can discover previously unknown primary or metastatic tumors, and, for some authors, can establish the SSTR status, clearly underlines its impact on patient management. This has been recently demonstrated in several series [23, 27, 40, 41].

The clinical impact of Octreoscan scintigraphy on management of patients with the ZES is high [23, 40] *(Table V)*.

Table V. Impact of Octreoscan scintigraphy on management of patients with the Zollinger-Ellison syndrome

Reference	Type of patients	Nb patients	Nb patients with impact on management (%)
[40]	All types of ZES	46	22 (47)
[23]	Sporadic ZES	39	19 (49)
[23]	MEN1+ZES	15	3 (20)
[23]	Liver metastases	14	4 (29)

In our group, the impact on management was lower in patients with ZES and MEN1 without liver metastases (20 %) than in patients with the sporadic type of the disease (49 %) [23]. Such a finding might be explained by our current therapeutic strategy in the ZES patients in whom a systematic surgical approach is offered only to sporadic ZES patients [42]. In patients with liver metastases, discovering controlateral metastases (when liver resection is contemplated) or extrahepatic metastases has a major impact on management, precluding surgery.

A recent preliminary study from the NIH conducted in 21 patients with sporadic ZES who had undergone surgery after Octreoscan scintigraphy, showed that the immediate postoperative cure rate did not differ from that in patients who had not undergone preoperative Octreoscan scintigraphy [25]. In our series of 21 patients with sporadic ZES who underwent surgery after Octreoscan scintigraphy, the immediate postoperative cure rate was also identical to that of the NIH patients who had not undergone preoperative Octreoscan scintigraphy [9]. This might suggest that, despite the fact that Octreoscan scintigraphy gives major additional information on the tumoral spread of the disease, it does not detect all the tumors and, therefore, does not increase the curative rate. This point remains to be confirmed by larger series.

In our entire series of 160 patients with different kinds of endocrine GEP tumors, Octreoscan modified patients' classification (presence or absence of hepatic and/or extrahepatic metastases) in 24 % of them and had an impact on surgical strategy in 25 % [41].

For some authors, the result of Octreoscan scintigraphy is considered a useful criteria to decide whether or not somatostatin therapy should be administered to an individual patient, especially in those with midgut carcinoids. Indeed, there is a good and significant global correlation between SSTR status and the effects of somatostatin analogs on peptide or amine levels [2, 6, 20, 30, 31]. However, in two recent series, discrepancies have been noted in 18 % to 20 % of the patients [30, 31]. When also considering the assessment of the SSTR status, Jamar et al. showed that Octreoscan scintigraphy provided information that guided the therapeutic decision in 20 (53 %) among 38 patients with different kinds of endocrine GEP tumors [27].

It has been suggested that a negative Octreoscan scintigraphy might indicate a poorly differentiated endocrine GEP tumor [43], since SSTR-negative carcinoids were often poorly differenciated [10]. It has also been shown that patients with a negative Octreoscan had a more malignant course, suggesting less differentiated tumors [31]. Since chemotherapy modalities in patients with metastatic undifferentiated tumors differ from those in patients with differentiated tumors, this information has been thought to be relevant [43].

Indications for Octreoscan scintigraphy in patients with endocrine gastroenteropancreatic tumors

In patients with (anatomically or biologically) proven endocrine GEP tumors, Octreoscan scintigraphy should be performed when an accurate evaluation of the tumoral spread is necessary, especially before surgery [9, 13, 22, 23, 27]. Before surgery, Octreoscan scintigraphy may give three types of information: 1- detection of previously unknown metastases that would contraindicate surgery; 2- detection of the primary tumor and the metastatic lymph nodes and 3- establishment of the SSTR status. Concerning the second point, as suggested recently in patients with the ZES, a better detection of the primary tumors with Octreoscan scintigraphy may not increase curability [25]. In patients with midgut carcinoids, the primary is often detected by the surgeon. Whether a better preoperative localization of the primary with Octreoscan scintigraphy increases the surgical detection rate remains to be determined in patients with midgut carcinoids, but this is likely. Concerning the third point, i.e., establishment of the SSTR status, the knowledge of a preoperative positive SSTR status is probably useful for the search for postoperative recurrence with Octreoscan.

When medical management is scheduled, we think that the indications of Octreoscan scintigraphy that would really modify management remain rather unclear [23]. In patients with liver metastases that could not be surgically treated (resection, transplantation), the detection of intra- or extraabdominal metastases with Octreoscan scintigraphy probably influences the treatment modalities, i.e., systemic treatments (chemotherapy, interferon, somatostatin analogs) will be prefered to localized treatment (liver chemoembolization).

Octreoscan scintigraphy seems extremely useful when there is a doubt on a potential endocrine tumor on conventional imaging (liver, pancreas or bone lesions, development of doubtful postoperative image).

Due to its cost, our opinion is that Octreoscan scintigraphy must not be performed exclusively in the attempt to determine SSTR status before initiating somatostatin analogue therapy. In this situation, measuring peptide or amine levels before and after acute administration of the somatostatin analog is probably more cost effective [22].

Finally, should Octreoscan scintigraphy be performed in the first-intention in the exploration of a patient with proven or suspected GEP tumors in order to reduce the number of other imaging techniques [24]? The answer is not currently available. However, from a pragmatic point of view, it must be remembered that, before the diagnosis of an endocrine tumor is suspected, most of the patients still have undergone many different investigations. Therefore, such a debate might be theoretical. In patients with the ZES, we and others think that both Octreoscan scintigraphy and endoscopic ultrasonography are the complementary techniques of choice [9, 13, 17, 28]. This is probably true for all types of pancreatic endocrine tumors.

Conclusion and perspectives

Octreoscan scintigraphy is the first efficient scintigraphy using labelled peptides in gastroenterological diseases. Due to its high sensitivity and specificity, as compared to other imaging techniques, Octreoscan scintigraphy is now commonly used in patients with endocrine GEP tumors. The impact of this technique on patient management seems high. The indications for Octreoscan scintigraphy are progressively more precise. However, prospective studies dealing with the impact of Octreoscan scintigraphy on patient management must still be extended. Binding labelled peptides to tumoral cells opens a large field of research: intraoperative detection of the tumors [44-46], radiotherapy [2], new peptides [47], or combination of different labelled somatostatin analogs.

References

1. Lamberts SWJ, Bakker WH, Reubi JC, Krenning EP. Somatostatin receptor imaging in the localization of endocrine tumours. *N Engl J Med* 1990; 323: 1246-9.
2. Krenning EP, Kwekkeboom DJK, Pauwels S, Kvols LK, Reubi JC. Somatostatin receptor scintigraphy. In: Freeman LM, ed. *Nuclear Medicine Annual.* New York: Raven Press Ltd 1995: 1-50.
3. Yamada Y, Post SR, Wang K, Tager HS, Bell GI, Seino S. Cloning and functional characterization of a family of human and mouse somatostatin receptors expressed in brain, gastrointestinal tract and kydney. *Proc Natl Acad Sci USA* 1992; 89: 251-5.
4. Yamada Y, Reisine S, Law SF, Ihara Y, Kubota A, Kagimoto S, Seino M, Seino Y, Bell GI, Seino S. Somatostatin receptors, an expanding gene family: cloning and functional characterization of human SSTR3, a protein coupled to adenylyl cyclase. *Mol Endocrinol* 1992; 6: 2136-42.
5. Yamada Y, Kagimoto S, Kubota A, Yasuka K, Masuda K, Someya Y, Ihara Y, Li Q, Imura H, Seino S, Seino Y. Cloning, functional expression and pharmacological characterization of a fourth

(hSSTR4) and a fifth (hSSTR5) human somatostatin receptor subtypes. *Biochem Biophys Res Commun* 1993; 195: 844-52.
6. Kubota A, Yamada Y, Kagimoto S, Shimatsu A, Imamura M, Tsuda K, Imura H, Seino S, Seino Y. Identification of somatostatin receptor subtypes and an implication for the efficacy of somatostatin analogue SMS 201-995 in treatment of human endocrine tumors. *J Clin Invest* 1994; 93: 1321-5.
7. John M, Meyerhof W, Richter D, Waser B, Schaer JC, Scherübl H, et al. Positive somatostatin receptor scintigraphy correlates with the presence of somatostatin receptor subtype 2. *Gut* 1996; 38: 33-9.
8. Krenning EP, Kwekkeboom DJ, Bakker WH, Breeman WAP, Kooij PPM, Oei HY, Van Hagen M, Postema PTE, De Jong M, Reubi JC, Visser TJ, Reijs AEM, Hofland LJ, Koper JW, Lamberts SWJ. Somatostatin receptor scintigraphy with [^{111}-In-DTPA-D-Phe^1]- and [^{123}I-Thyr^3]-octreotide: the Rotterdam experience with more than 1000 patients. *Eur J Nucl Med* 1993; 20: 716-31.
9. Cadiot G, Lebtahi R, Sarda L, Bonnaud G, Marmuse JP, Vissuzaine C, Ruszniewski P, Le Guludec D, Mignon M, GRESZE. Preoperative detection of duodenal gastrinomas and peripancreatic lymph nodes by somatostatin receptor scintigraphy. *Gastroenterology* 1996 (in press).
10. Reubi JC, Kvols LK, Waser B, Nagorney D, Heitz PU, Charboneau JW, Reading CC, Moertel C. Detection of somatostatin receptors in surgical and percutaneous needle biopsy samples of carcinoids and islet cell carcinomas. *Cancer Res* 1990; 50: 5969-77.
11. Reubi JC, Horisberger U, Essed CE, Jeekel J, Klijn JGH, Lamberts SWJ. Absence of somatostatin receptors in human exocrine pancreatic adenocarcinomas. *Gastroenterology* 1988; 95: 760-3.
12. Krenning EP, Bakker WH, Kooij PPM, Breeman WAP, Oei HY, De Jong M, Reubi JC, Visser TJ, Bruns C, Kwekkeboom DJ, Reijs AEM, Van Hagen PM, Koper JW, Lamberts SWJ. Somatostatin receptor scintigraphy with [^{111}-In-DTPA-D-Phe^1]-octreotide in man: metabolism, dosimetry and comparison with [^{123}I-Thyr^3]-octreotide. *J Nucl Med* 1992; 33: 652-8.
13. De Kerviler E, Cadiot G, Lebtahi R, Faraggi M, Le Guludec D, Mignon M, GRESZE. Somatostatin receptor scintigraphy in forty-eight patients with the Zollinger-Ellison syndrome. *Eur J Nucl Med* 1994; 21: 1191-7.
14. Dörr U, Räth U, Sautter-Bihl M-L, Guzman G, Bach D, Adrian H-J, Bihl H. Improved visualization of carcinoid liver metastases by indium-^{111}-Pentetreotide scintigraphy following treatment with cold somatostatin analogue. *Eur J Nucl Med* 1993; 20: 431-3.
15. Lebtahi R, Petegnief Y, Cadiot G, Sarda L, Daou D, Mignon M, Faraggi M, Le Guludec D. Additional value of SPECT in the detection of gastro-entero-pancreatic (GEP) tumors with somatostatin receptor scintigraphy (SRS) (Abstract). *J Nucl Med* 1996; 37: 256P-7P.
16. Ur E, Bomanji J, Mather SJ, Britton KE, Wass JAH, Grossman AB, Besser GM. Localization of neuroendocrine tumours and insulinomas using radiolabelled somatostatin analogues, ^{123}I-Thyr^3-octreotide and ^{111}-In-Pentatreotide. *Clin Endocrinol* 1993; 38: 501-6.
17. Zimmer T, Ziegler K, Bäder M, Fett U, Hamm B, Riecken EO, Wiedenmann. Localisation of neuroendocrine tumours of the upper gastrointestinal tract. *Gut* 1994; 35: 471-5.
18. Scherübl H, Bäder M, Fett U, Hamm B, Schmidt-Gayk H, Koppenhagen K, Dop F-J, Reicken E-O, Wiedenmann B. Somatostatin-receptor imaging of neuroendocrine gastroenteropancreatic tumors. *Gastroenterology* 1993; 103: 1705-9.
19. Kwekkeboom DJ, Krenning EP, Bakker WH, Oei HY, Kooij PPM, Lamberts SWJ. Somatostatin analogue scintigraphy in carcinoid tumours. *Eur J Nucl Med* 1993; 20: 283-92.
20. Kvols LK, Brown ML, O'Connor MK, Hung JC, Hayostek RJ, Reubi JC, Lamberts SWJ. Evaluation of a radiolabeled somatostatin analog (I-123 Octreotide) in the detection and localization of carcinoid and islet cell tumors. *Radiology* 1993; 187: 129-33.
21. Joseph K, Stapp J, Reinecke J, Skamel HJ, Höffken H, Neuhaus Ch, Lenze H, Trautman ME, Arnold R. ^{111}-In-Pentetreotide receptor scintigraphy in neuroendocrine gastroenteropancreatic tumors. *Horm Metab Res* 1993; 27 (Suppl): 28-35.

22. Carnaille B, Nocaudie M, Pattou F, Huglo D, Deveaux M, Marchandise X, Proye C. Scintiscans and carcinoid tumors. *Surgery* 1994; 116: 1118-22.
23. Bonnaud G, Cadiot G, Lebtahi R, Sarda L, Le Guludec D, Mignon M. Clinical implications of Octreoscan scintigraphy in 68 patients with the Zollinger-Ellison syndrome (ZES) (Abstract). *Gastroenterology* 1996; 110: A380.
24. Gibril F, Reynolds JC, Doppman JL, Chen CC, Venzon DJ, Termanini B, Weber HC, Stewart CA, Jensen RT. Somatostatin receptor scintigraphy: its sensitivity compared with that of other imaging methods in detecting primary and metastatic gastrinomas. A prospective study. *Ann Intern Med* 1996; 125: 26-34.
25. Gibril F, Fraker DL, Alexander HR, Termanini B, Stewart CA, Sutliff VE, Jensen RT. Does the use of preoperative somatostatin receptor scintigraphy (SRS) have an impact in improving postoperative cure rate in patients undergoing surgery with Zollinger-Ellison syndrome (ZES): a prospective study (Abstract). *Gastroenterology* 1996; 110: A391.
26. Schirmer WJ, Melvin WS, Rush RM, O'Dorisio TM, Pozderac RV, Olsen JO, Ellison EC. Indium-[111]-Pentetreotide scanning versus conventional imaging techniques for the localization of gastrinoma. *Surgery* 1995; 118: 1105-14.
27. Jamar F, Fiasse R, Leners N, Pauwels S. Somatostatin receptor imaging with Indium-[111]-Pentetreotide in gastroenteropancreatic neuroendocrine tumors: safety, efficacy and impact on patient management. *J Nucl Med* 1995; 36: 542-9.
28. Zimmer T, Liehr RM, Stötzel U, Fett U, Bäder M, Riecken EO, Wiedenmann B. Endoscopic ultrasonography (EUS) and somatostatin-receptor-scintigraphy (SRS) for the localization of insulinomas and gastrinomas. *Gastroenterology* 1994; 106: A331.
29. Westlin J-E, Janson ET, Ahlström H, Nilsson S, Öhrvall U, Öberg K. Scintigraphy using [111]-Indium-labeled somatostatin analogue for localization of neuroendocrine tumors. *Antibody, Immunoconjugates, and Radiopharmaceuticals* 1992; 5: 367-84.
30. Nocaudie-Calzada M, Huglo D, Deveaux M, Carnaille B, Proye C, Marchandise X. Iodine-123-Tyr-3-Octreotide uptake in pancreatic endocrine tumors and in carcinoids in relation to hormonal inhibition by octreotide. *J Nucl Med* 1994; 35: 57-62.
31. Tiensuu Janson E, Westlin J-E, Eriksson B, Ahlström H, Nilsso, S, Öberg K. [[111]-In-DTPA-D-Phe[1]] Octreotide scintigraphy in patients with carcinoid tumours: the predictive value for somatostatin analogue treatment. *Eur J Endocrinol* 1994; 131: 577-81.
32. Krenning EP, Kwekkeboom DJ, Oei HY, de Jong RJB, Dop FJ, de Herder WW, Reubi JC, Lamberts SWJ. Somatostatin receptor scintigraphy in carcinoids, gastrinomas and Cushing's syndrome. *Digestion* 1994; 55 (suppl 3): 54-9.
33. Kälkner K-M, Tiensuu Janson E, Nilsson S, Carlsson S, Öberg K, Westlin J-E. Somatostatin receptor scintigraphy in patients with carcinoid tumors: comparison between radioligand uptake and tumor markers. *Cancer Res* 1995; 55 (suppl.): 5801s-4s.
34. Termanini B, Gibril F, Doppman JH, Stewart CA, Sutliff VE, Jensen RT. Somatostatin receptor scintigraphy (SRS), a new method to distinguish hepatic hemangiomas from vascular liver metastases in pancreatic endocrine tumors (PET) (Abstract). *Gastroenterology* 1996; 110: A437.
35. Orbuch M, Doppman JL, Strader DB, Fishbeyn VA, Benya RV, Metz DC, Jensen RT. Imaging for pancreatic endocrine tumor localization: recent advances. In: Mignon M, Jensen RT eds. *Endocrine tumors of the pancreas. Recent advances in research and management.* Basel: Karger, 1995; 23: 268-81.
36. Ruszniewski Ph, Amouyal P, Amouyal G, Grangé JD, Mignon M, Bouché O, Bernades P. Localization of gastrinomas by endoscopic ultrasonography in patients with Zollinger-Ellison syndrome. *Surgery* 1995; 117: 629-35.
37. Cadiot G, Lebtahi R, Faraggi M, Le Guludec D, Mignon M. Detection of bone metastases of endocrine tumors: comparison of somatostatin receptor scintigraphy with bone scintigraphy: preliminary results (Abstract). *Gastroenterology* 1995; 108: A346.

38. Gibril F, Termanini B, Stewart CA, Sutliff VE, Jensen RT. Prospective study of the occurrence of metastases to bone in patients with Zollinger-Ellison syndrome (ZES) (Anstract). *Gastroenterology* 1996; 110: A1073.
39. Modlin IM, Cornelius E, Lawton GP. Use of an isotopic somatostatin receptor probe to image gut endocrine tumors. *Arch Surg* 1995; 130: 367-74.
40. Gibril F, Reynolds JC, Doppman JL, Chen CC, Termanini B, Stewart CA, Jensen RT. Does the use of octreoscanning alter management in patients with Zollinger-Ellison syndrome: a prospective study? (Abstract). *Gastroenterology* 1995; 108: A194.
41. Lebtahi R, Cadiot G, Sarda L, Daou D, Faraggi M, Marmuse JP, Delahaye N, Mignon M, Le Guludec D. Somatostatin receptor scintigraphy in gastroenteropancreatic (GEP) tumors: therapeutic implications (Abstract). *J Nucl Med* 1996; 37: 253P.
42. Mignon M, Cadiot G, Rigaud D, Ruszniewski P, Jaïs P, Lehy T, Lewin MJM. The management of islet cell tumors in patients with multiple endocrine neoplasia type 1 (MEN 1). In: Mignon M, Jensen RT, eds. *Endocrine tumors of the pancreas: recent advances in research and management.* Basel: Karger, 1995; 23: 342-59.
43. Reubi JC. Clinical relevance of somatostatin receptor imaging. *Eur J Endocrinol* 1994; 131: 575-6.
44. Cadiot G, Lebtahi R, Marmuse JP, Le Guludec D, Mignon M. Prospective evaluation of intraoperative isotopic detection of gastrinomas after ^{111}-In-Pentetreotide administration: preliminary results in 5 patients (Abstract). *Gastroenterology* 1996; 110: A381.
45. Schirmer WJ, O'Dorisio TM, Schirmer TP, Mojzisik CM, Hinkle GH, Martin EW. Intraoperative localization of neuroendocrine tumors with 125-TYR(3)-octreotide and a hand-held-gamma-detecting probe. *Surgery* 1993; 114: 745-52.
46. Wängberg B, Forssell-Aronsson E, Tisell LE, Nilsson O, Fjälling M, Ahlman H. Intraoperative detection of somatostatin-receptor-positive neuroendocrine tumours using indium-^{111}-labelled DTPA-D-Phe1-octreotide. *Br J Cancer* 1996; 73: 770-5.
47. Virgolini I, Raderer M, Kurtaran A, Angelberger P, Banyal S, Yang, Q, Li S, Banyai M, Pidlich J, Nierdele B, Scheithauer W, Valent P. Vasoactive intestinal peptide-receptor imaging for the localization of intestinal adenocarcinomas and endocrine tumors. *N Engl J Med* 1994; 331: 1116-21.

Progress in the treatment of liver metastases

T. Sauerbruch, R. Caspari, T. Heinicke, J. Metzger

Department of General Internal Medicine, University of Bonn, FRG

Summary

Liver metastases due to intestinal primaries signify in most patients a dismal prognosis. Only a small number of these has any chance of a cure. These are either patients with endocrine tumors or patients with secondaries from colorectal carcinoma. In Europe, the age-adjusted incidence of colorectal cancer is around 50 cases/100,000 population/year. At time of diagnosis, 15-25 % of the patients have synchronous liver metastases. After curative resection, recurrent metastatic disease occurs in 20-50 % of the patients. However, in only 5 % of these patients will disease be limited to the liver. Furthermore, only a small percentage of patients with liver metastases and no secondaries outside the liver are treated successfully, primarily by surgical resection. Regional chemotherapy (e.g. using 5-fluoro-2-desoxyuridine or 5-fluorouracil) can be applied in patients who do not qualify for hepatic resection. Since the liver is rarely the sole site of dissemination, systematic chemotherapy using 5-fluorouracil with or without different modulators such as leucovorin is most often applied. All these treatments have a response rate in the range of 20-50 %. Yet, the impact on life-prolongation is small. The future will show whether new chemotherapy modalities, immunotherapy or gene therapy can prolong a patient's life-span and offer an acceptable quality of life.

Secondary hepatic malignancy in most cases is blood borne with primaries in the intestine – mainly the colorectum –, in the stomach or in the pancreas. However, lung cancer, breast cancer, kidney or adrenal neoplasias, less often uterus cancer, ovarian cancer or melanoma may also disseminate to the liver, which is the largest human parenchymal organ.

Liver metastases almost always are a sign of advanced malignant disease indicating a fatal outcome for most patients within less than 1-2 years [1]. Thus, therapy should focus on palliation, *i.e.* the alleviation of pain or relief from obstructive jaundice, if possible. In a limited number of patients, treatment of liver metastases can aim at a prolongation of life or even a cure. The percentage of these candidates, however, is extremely low. Such patients are almost exclusively those with primaries in the colon and rectum or with endocrine tumors and few patients with breast cancer as well as small cell lung cancer. These patients should be filtered out from the vast majority of those with a pessimistic prognosis. It is critical that – prior to treatment – disseminated disease outside the liver is ruled out by diagnosic approaches such as contrast enhanced computed tomography, magnetic resonance imaging (MRI), or even positron emission tomography (PET). A systematic staging is also mandatory to allow exact classification and comparable documentation [2] *(Table I)*.

Table I. Check list for evaluation of patients with liver metastases and colorectal carcinoma

a)	Date of diagnosis of colorectal carcinoma.
b)	Location, histological type and grade of primary tumor.
c)	Date of diagnosis of liver metastases and of histological confirmation. Histological type and grade.
d)	Location of metastases according to the segmental anatomy of Couinauld, number of metastases and size including the diagnostic method, percentage of liver involvement, involvement of intrahepatic vessels, involvement of adjacent structures.
e)	Diagnostic steps to assess or rule out extrahepatic tumor manifestation including the primary tumor, lymph nodes, lungs and bones, etc.
f)	Other clinical findings: - symptoms and signs (jaundice, pain, weight loss, hepatomegaly), - pathological liver function tests, - concomitant liver disease such as hepatitis or cirrhosis, - Karnofsky status, - dynamic growth of liver metastases if possible (*e.g.* doubling time), - assessment of operative risk according to the ASA criteria.

The present paper focusses on liver metastases caused by primary colorectal carcinoma that permit classical and less classical therapeutic possibilities. About 15-25 % of patients with newly diagnosed colorectal carcinoma have synchronous hepatic metastases. On the other hand, in 80 % of patients with distant colorectal carcinoma, the liver is involved [3]. According to retrospective analyses, median survival in patients with liver metastases without therapeutic intervention may be around 10 months, ranging from 3 to 24 months [1].

After excluding extrahepatic metastases by a thorough evaluation of the patient, several therapeutic options exist, *i.e.* hepatic resection, regional chemotherapy, different modalities of systemic chemotherapy, regional injection of necrosing substances such as alcohol, immunomodulatory therapy with or without concomitant chemotherapy or radiotherapy. In addition, phase I/II gene therapeutic trials have recently been started.

Hepatic resection

After a careful diagnostic workup with special emphasis on exclusion of local, regional and distant extrahepatic recurrences, only a small percentage of patients qualifies for liver resection. These are patients in a good general condition with other favourable prognostic signs, who have no more than three (in selected cases four) independent metastases in the liver. Intraoperative hepatic ultrasound is important to assess the exact number of metastatic nodules as well as their anatomical location and to rule out further occult nodules not assessed by preoperative staging. According to a large prospective evaluation, nearly half of the patients scheduled for liver resection can have curative resection, about 10 % non-curative resection while 40 % are found to be unresectable [4].

Patients with synchronous metastases to the liver are believed to have a worse prognosis than patients with recurrent disease after curative resection of the primary tumor. However, in only 5-8 % of the patients, recurrent disease is confined to the liver. In these cases hepatic involvement shows lesions limited to the left lobe in 10-15 % of patients, to the right lobe in 20-40 % and to both lobes in 50-70 % of the patients [3].

The operative mortality of liver resection averages 5 %, with postoperative complications (subphrenic abscess, intraabdominal bleeding, bile leak, hepatic failure, coagulopathies, pulmonary complications, wound infections or deep vein thrombosis) ranging between 15 and 40 % [1]. After resection, prognosis is determined by several factors, the relevance of which is somewhat controversial. Factors believed to indicate a bad prognosis include the number of four or more metastases, size of metastases (> 4 cm), mesenteric lymph node involvement, limited resection margins (< 1 cm), bilobular liver disease, poor differentiation of primary tumor (grade III/IV), non-anatomic resection, disease free survival less than one year after resection of the primary tumor, and concomitant liver disease such as cirrhosis or hepatitis [3, 5, 6].

Five-year actuarial survival rates between 20 % and 40 % after surgery can be achieved in carefully selected patients. However, the percentage of patients with disease free survival is considerably smaller. The percentages of patients surviving five years are better than those known from historical controls not operated upon. However, it is not quite clear whether the median survival time is really positively influenced. Patients in good general condition with solitary metastases smaller than 4 cm fare best, however, they constitute only a small minority. In some of these, a cure may be realized.

Since most patients cannot be saved by resection, the question as to whether adjuvant chemotherapy should be performed has been risen [7]. Yet, the role of adjuvant chemotherapy after resection is ill-defined to date. Preliminary small trials suggest that some patients profit from adjuvant treatment, that uses local or systemic chemotherapy [8].

After curative resection, about 75 % of patients will suffer recurrent disease within five years [9]. A small percentage of these patients might again qualify for liver surgery. However, a current series on repeated hepatectomy is small [10]. The operation takes longer, is technically more demanding and accompanied by a higher amount of blood loss. Long-term survival after repeated resection for colorectal secondaries is extremely rare [11]. Therefore, other techniques such as local alcohol injection or even cryosurgery have to be considered [12, 13].

Regional chemotherapy

Regional chemotherapy can be applied in patients who do not qualify for hepatic resection and who do not have extrahepatic disease. The local intrahepatic infusion of chemotherapy agents has the advantage that considerably higher drug levels are achieved at the site of metastatic disease along with less systemic toxicity, especially if substances with a high hepatic extraction rate are used.

Regional chemotherapy is based on the fact that hepatic metastases are mainly supplied by arterial vessels, whereas normal liver tissue receives its major nutrition *via* portal-venous blood [14]. Usually, a catheter is placed in the gastroduodenal artery with the tip at the junction with the hepatic artery [1]. In order to prevent an inadvertent application of the drug to extrahepatic organs such as the duodenum or the stomach, particular care has to be taken to identify an aberrant hepatic arterial system and to divert those vessels distal from the catheter's tip that allow perfusion of the stomach and duodenum. Furthermore, dislodgement of the catheter should be prevented. In summary, catheter implantation requires experience and skill.

Although the liver receives an increased exposure with respect to systemic levels that ranges between 2-5 fold (cisplatinum and mitomycin) and 50-100 fold (5-fluoro-2-desoxyuridine, 5-FUDR, 5-fluorouracil, 5-FU), the absolute systemic exposure resembles the standard i.v. route, with the exception of 5-FUDR, which has by far the highest hepatic extraction rate [1, 15]. The administration of intrahepatic FUDR leads to a response rate of around 50 % [16, 17], which in most randomized trials has been higher than that of an i.v. systemic therapy using 5-FUDR or 5-FU with a response rate of 10-20 %. However, these favourable results have not translated into prolonged survival, because of several important drawbacks: a relatively high *de novo* resistance to FUDR or its combinations, an acquired resistance after initial response, extrahepatic tumor progression, or damage due to the bile duct toxicity of FUDR [18, 19]. Furthermore, intrahepatic treatment is expensive and should be restricted to experts. Although some of these drawbacks could be diminished by reducing the FUDR dose and modifying the application schedule, by improving the catheter and port devices, by checking the perfusion of substances prior to drug application with radionuclide methods or by combining local FUDR instillation with dexamethasone [17], some major concerns remain. In the light of the new rather effective systemic therapy using continuous 5-FU infusion together with leucovorin [20-22], it may be cheaper, less troublesome for the patient and more effective against extrahepatic disease to start with systemic chemotherapy and to restrict local therapy to patients who have failed systemic therapy and still have metastatic disease restricted to the liver [18, 19]. In these patients, FUDR is one of the choices. However, other modalities such as chemoembolisation with lipiodol and 5-FU, IFN alfa 2a and anthracyclins or chemo-biotherapy regimens can also be considered [23-25]. Local therapy using 5-FU alone or in combination with folinic acid leads to a high drug concentration in the liver together with adequate systemic drug levels and is worth consideration [26]. The combination of local chemotherapy and systemic chemotherapy at the same time has only been systematically studied in small patient series [27].

Systemic therapy

Systemic chemotherapy is most frequently used in patients with colorectal carcinoma and hepatic metastases, mainly due to the fact that in the majority of patients the liver is not the sole site of dissemination. Since the mid-1950s the main-stay of therapy has been 5-FU. Response rates obtained with standard bolus regimens range between 10 and 20 %. Since then significant progress has been made with respect to 5-FU based regimens in terms of modulation with other substances, dosage or time schedule [28].

The different modulators and their mode of action are listed in *Table II*. The most important substance is leucovorin, a reduced folate that enhances the cytotoxicity of 5-FU by increasing FdUMP which is an inhibitor of thymidylate synthase. Several trials have shown that 5-FU combined with leucovorin is superior to 5-FU alone, especially if classical 5-day regimens of 5-FU every four weeks were used. Leucovorin is given at a low dosage (20 mg/m^2 over 5 days) or a high dosage (200 mg/m^2 over 5 days or 500 mg/m^2 weekly) prior to 5-FU [21, 29]. This improved response rate, however, did again not translate into an improved survival rate. This is mainly due to the low rate of complete remissions (< 5 %) [16]. At the moment, a study is under way that compares continuous infusion of 5-FU (2,6 g/m^2/24 h) at weekly intervals with or without modulators such as leucovorin or N-phosphonacetyl-L-aspartate (PALA) *versus* the classical 5-day schedule every four weeks [16].

Table II. Biochemical modulation of 5-FU therapy in patients with advanced colorectal cancer

Biochemical modulator	Dosage	Mode of action	Improvement of the response rate in randomized trials
Leucovorin	Low 20 mg/m^2, 5d High 200 mg/m^2, 5d [29]	Stabilization of the ternary complex of FdUMP, N^5 M^{10} methylene-FH$_4$, and thymidilate synthase [20]	+
Methotrexate	40-500 mg/m^2 [31]	Inhibition of purine synthesis leading to increased FUTP levels [31]	+
PALA (N-(phosphonacetyl)-L-aspartate	250 mg/m^2 [35, 45]	Depletion of various nucleotides, inhibition of RNA synthesis [45]	Not tested
Alfa-2a-interferon	10 MU three times weekly [33, 34]	Increased FdUMP levels and incorporation into DNA, prolonged *in vivo*-half-life of 5-FU [34, 46, 47]	-

The question as to whether treatment should be initiated in the asymptomatic patient or only in case of symptomatic disease is important, especially in consideration of the fact that all these patients eventually die and that the burden of treatment should not decrease life quality. One study [30] showed that early treatment prolonged survival by about five months as compared to a group in which treatment was instituted only in case of symptomatic disease.

Bolus treatment mainly causes bone marrow suppression (~14 %) and stomatitis (~13 %), whereas under continuous infusion, leukopenia and stomatitis occur in less than 5 % of patients, but hand-foot-syndrome occurs in every fourth patient. 5-FU can rarely also aggravate coronary heart disease by causing vasospasm.

Modulation of 5-FU treatment with methotrexate [31] increases the response rate to 5-FU from approximately 10 % to 20 % (complete response from 2 % to 3 %). The interval between methotrexate and 5-FU should be longer than four hours. The role of leucovorin rescue in the results of these trials is not clear at the moment. The survival benefit of methotrexate modulation was modest, if present at all.

In vitro studies have shown that the recombinant interferon alfa 2a or - alfa 2b increases the formation of the active metabolite fluorodesoxyuridinemonophosphate and enhances the incorporation of the active metabolite into the DNA. Therefore interferon has been suggested as a response modifier of 5-FU [32, 33]. According to a randomized trial, interferon at a dosage of 10 millions three times a week enhances toxicity causing leukopenia, lymphopenia, depression and alopecia without any additional benefit [34].

A recent paper has questioned a major impact of modulation on 5-FU treatment [35]. Hopefully, new drugs such as camptothecins [36] will have a further and more potent impact on systemic treatment of advanced colorectal disease. Experimental data is promising.

Immunotherapy

The concept of inducing or augmenting a specific immunoreaction of the host against the tumor has been pursued for nearly a century. Two strategies are evaluated, activation of cytolytic lymphocytes (CTL), which are restricted by the HLA I system, and adoptive immunotherapy with activated natural killer (A-NK) cells, which are non-MHC restricted and recognize tumor cells without prior sensitization.

Active specific immunotherapy uses Newcastle disease virus infected autologous tumor cells to increase CTL response. The epitopes against which the cellular immunoresponse is directed remains unclear. Preliminary studies have shown that active specific immunotherapy may increase the rate of disease free survival after RO-resection of hepatic metastases [37]. Experience, however, is very limited. Experience with IL-2 stimulated natural killer cells is even more limited [38]. A number of problems remain to be solved, such as identification of the epitopes, degree of cellular infiltration at the tumor site (probably less than 5-10 % of intravenous transferred cells), bystander effects, clinical relevance, etc.

New approaches must also adopt new molecular genetic methods such as transfection of genes into autologous tumor cells that encode costimulatory surface molecules such as B7 *(see Gene therapy)*. To date, it is unclear whether these immunotherapeutic approaches are able to provide significant improvement of the therapy of advanced colorectal cancer.

Probably, their value may be highest in the adjuvant situation where micrometastases cannot be ruled out. It is intriguing that this therapy has no chemical toxicity.

Gene therapy

Gene therapy for liver metastases could envisage direct action on tumor cells to induce drug sensitization or enhancement of immunorecognition of malignant cells. Theoretically, there are several possibilities to introduce prodrug-activating genes into tumor cells. Incorporation of the herpes simplex virus thymidine kinase (TK) gene into dividing tumor cells, *e.g.* by retroviral vectors, leads to the synthesis of a cytotoxic nucleotide after application of ganciclovir [39]. Furthermore, animal studies, using a colorectal carcinoma cell-line showed that the prodrug 5-fluorocytosine (FCyt) can be metabolized to the toxic 5-fluorouracil (5-FU) within the cells after retroviral vector delivery of a gene into these cells that encodes the enzyme cytosine deaminase [40]. Genes which lead to expression of immunoactivating surface molecules, such as B7-1 (CD80) or B7-2 (CD86) or cytokines may also be transferred into malignant cells, enhancing their immunogenicity [41, 42].

To date, however, several major obstacles exist: sufficient gene engraftment onto the tumor cells – especially if retroviral vectors are used – is probably not feasible because only dividing cells are reached. The problem can be solved by using adenoviral vectors. However, genes delivered by this system do not integrate into the genome of the host cell. They are gradually lost by cell division. Immunological reaction against viral proteins is a further problem, yet may enhance tumor cell killing by CTL. Specificity of expression in tumor cells, which is important, can be achieved by creating a chimeric gene composed of a tumor cell specific promoter (*e.g.* from the CEA-gene) and a cDNA sequence encoding the therapeutic protein. Some of the problems of gene therapy are probably more easily solved by *ex vivo* targeting [39, 43]. Phase I-trials are under way to test the feasibility in man.

Miscellaneous new approaches

Ultrasound-guided percutaneous alcohol injection [12], intraoperative high dose radiation [44] or percutaneous irradiation are further approaches to liver metastases, the natural history of which is difficult to influence.

Acknowledgement
We thank Mrs Sylvia Körner for superb secretarial help.

References

1. Niederhuber JE, Ensminger WD. Treatment of metastatic cancer. In: DeVita VT jr, Hellman S, Rosenberg SA, eds. *Cancer - Principles and practice of oncology*. 4th Edition. Philadelphia: JB Lippincott Company, 1993: 2201-25.

2. Wittekind C. Klassifikation und Dokumentation von Lebermetastasen kolorektaler Karzinome. *Zentralbl Chir* 1995; 120: 760-3.
3. Ballantyne GH, Quin J. Surgical treatment of liver metastases in patients with colorectal cancer. *Cancer* 1993; 71: 4252-66.
4. Steele G, Bleday R, Mayer RJ, Lindblad A, Petrelli N, Weaver D. A prospective evaluation of hepatic resection for colorectal carcinoma metastases to the liver: gastrointestinal tumor study group protocol 6584. *J Clin Oncol* 1991; 9: 1105-12.
5. Pedersen IK, Burcharth F, Roikjaer O, Baden H. Resection of liver metastases from colorectal cancer. *Dis Colon Rectum* 1994; 37: 1078-82.
6. Scheele J, Stangl R, Altendorf-Hofmann A, Gall FP. Indicators of prognosis after hepatic resection for colorectal secondaries. *Surgery* 1991; 110: 13-29.
7. de Jong KP, Slooff MJH, de Vries EGE, Brouwers MAM, Terpstra OT. Effect of partial liver resection on tumour growth. *J Hepatol* 1996; 25: 109-21.
8. Lorenz M, Staib-Sebler E, Rossion I, Koch B, Cog C, Encke A. Ergebnisse der Resektion und adjuvanten Therapie von Lebermetastasen kolorektaler Primärtumoren - eine Literaturübersicht. *Zentralbl Chir* 1995; 120: 769-79.
9. Greenway B. Hepatic metastases from colorectal cancer: resection or not. *Br J Surg* 1988; 75: 513-9.
10. Elias D, Lasser Ph, Hoang JM, Leclere J, Debaene B, Bognel C, Spencer A, Rougier Ph. Repeat hepatectomy for cancer. *Br J Surg* 1993; 80: 1557-62.
11. Nordlinger B, Vaillant JCh, Guiguet M, Balladur P, Paris F, Bachellier Ph, Jaeck D and the Association Francaise de Chirurgie. Survival benefit of repeat liver resections for recurrent colorectal metastases: 143 cases. *J Clin Oncol* 1994; 12: 1491-6.
12. Giovannini M, Seitz J-F. Ultrasound-guided percutaneous alcohol injection of small liver metastases. *Cancer* 1994; 73: 294-7.
13. Ravikumar TS, Steele G, Kane R, King V. Experimental and clinical observations on hepatic cryosurgery for colorectal metastases. *Cancer Res* 1991; 51: 6323-7.
14. Strohmeyer T, Haugeberg G, Lierse W. Angioarchitecture and blood supply of micro- and macrometastases in human livers. *J Hepatol* 1987; 4: 181-9.
15. Schalhorn A, Kühl M. Pharmakologie der regionalen Chemotherapie kolorektaler Lebermetastasen. *Zentralbl Chir* 1995; 120: 764-8.
16. Vaughn DJ, Haller DG. Nonsurgical management of recurrent colorectal cancer. *Cancer* 1993; 71: 4278-92.
17. Kemeny NE. Is hepatic infusion of chemotherapy effective treatment for liver metastases? Yes! *Important Adv Oncol* 1992: 207-27.
18. Patt YZ. Regional hepatic arterial chemotherapy for colorectal cancer metastatic to the liver: the controversy continues (editorial). *J Clin Oncol* 1993; 11: 815-9.
19. O'Connell MJ. Is hepatic infusion of chemotherapy effective treatment for liver metastases? No! *Important Adv Oncol* 1992: 229-34.
20. Ardalan B, Chua L, Tian E, Reddy R, Sridhar K, Benedetto P, Richman S, Legaspi A, Waldman S, Morrell L, Feun L, Savaraj N, Livingstone A. A phase II study of weekly 24-hour infusion with high-dose fluorouracil with leucovorin in colorectal carcinoma. *J Clin Oncol* 1991; 9: 625-30.
21. Buroker TR, O'Connell MJ, Wieand HS, Krook JE, Gerstner JB, Mailliard JA, Schaefer PL, Levitt R, Kardinal CG, Gesme DH. Randomized comparison of two schedules of fluorouracil and leucovorin in the treatment of advanced colorectal cancer. *J Clin Oncol* 1994; 12: 14-20.
22. Grem JL, Jordan E, Robson ME, Binder RA, Hamilton JM, Steinberg SM, Arbuck SG, Beveridge RA, Kales AN, Miller JA, Weiss RB, McAtee N, Chen A, Goldspiel B, Sover E, Allegra CJ. Phase II study of fluorouracil, leucovorin, and interferon alfa-2a in metastatic colorectal carcinoma. *J Clin Oncol* 1993; 11: 1737-45.

23. Martinelli DJ, Wadler S, Bakal CW, Cynamon J, Rozenblit A, Haynes H, Kaleya R, Wiernik PH. Utility of embolization or chemoembolization as second-line treatment in patients with advanced or recurrent colorectal carcinoma. *Cancer* 1994; 74: 1706-12.
24. Lang EK, Brown ChL. Colorectal metastases to the liver: selective chemoembolisation. *Radiology* 1993; 189: 417-22.
25. Görich J, Hasan I, Sittek H, Kunze V, Gallkowski U, Majdali R, Müller-Miny H, Mezger I, Hartlapp JH, Reiser M, Steudel A. Embolisation von primären und sekundären Lebertumoren. *Radiologia Diagnostica* 1993; 34: 289-303.
26. Staib-Sebler E, Lorenz M, Gog C, Encke A. Continuous arterial 5-fluorouracil and folinic acid chemotherapy for colorectal liver metastases. *Onkologie* 1995; 18: 240-4.
27. Kemeny N, Conti JA, Sigurdson E, Cohen A, Seiter K, Lincer R, Niedzwiecki D, Botet J, Chapman D, Costa P, Budd A. A pilot study of hepatic artery floxuridine combined with systemic 5-fluorouracil and leucovorin. *Cancer* 1993; 71: 1964-71.
28. Moertel CG. Chemotherapy for colorectal cancer. *N Engl J Med* 1994; 330: 1136-42.
29. Poon MA, O'Connell MJ, Wieand HS, Krook JE, Gerstner JB, Tschetter LK, Levitt R, Kardinal CG, Mailliard JA. Biochemical modulation of fluorouracil with leucovorin: confirmatory evidence of improved therapeutic efficacy in advanced colorectal cancer. *J Clin Oncol* 1991; 9: 1967-72.
30. The Nordic Gastrointestinal Tumor Adjuvant Therapy Group. Expectancy or primary chemotherapy in patients with advanced asymptomatic colorectal cancer: a randomized trial. *J Clin Oncol* 1992; 10: 904-11.
31. The Advanced Colorectal Cancer Meta-Analysis Project. Meta-analysis of randomized trials testing the biochemical modulation of fluorouracil by methotrexate in metastatic colorectal cancer. *J Clin Oncol* 1994; 12: 960-9.
32. Wadler S, Wersto R, Weinberg V, Thompson D, Schwartz EL. Interaction of fluorouracil and interferon in human colon cancer cell lines: cytotoxic and cytokinetic effects. *Cancer Res* 1990; 50: 5735-9.
33. Wadler S, Lembersky B, Atkins M, Kirkwood J, Petrelli N. Phase II trial of fluorouracil and recombinant interferon alfa-2a in patients with advanced colorectal carcinoma: an Eastern cooperative oncology group study. *J Clin Oncol* 1991; 9: 1806-10.
34. Hill M, Norman A, Cunningham D, Findlay M, Nicolson V, Hill A, Iveson A, Evans Ch, Joffe J, Nicolson M, Hickish T. Royal Marsden phase III trial of fluorouracil with or without interferon alfa-2b in advanced colorectal cancer. *J Clin Oncol* 1995; 13: 1297-302.
35. Leichman CG, Fleming TR, Muggia FM, Tangen CM, Ardalan B, Doroshow JH, Meyers FJ, Holcombe RF, Weiss GR, Mangalik A, Macdonald JS. Phase II study of fluorouracil and its modulation in advanced colorectal cancer: a Southwest oncology group study. *J Clin Oncol* 1995; 13: 1303-11.
36. Potmesil M, Vardeman D, Kozielski AJ, Mendoza J, Stehlin JS, Giovanella BC. Growth inhibition of human cancer metastases by camptothecins in newly developed xenograft models. *Cancer Res* 1995; 55: 5637-41.
37. Hagmüller E, Beck N, Ockert D, Schirrmacher V. Adjuvante Therapie von Lebermetastasen. Aktive spezifische Immuntherapie. *Zentrabl Chir* 1995; 120: 780-5.
38. Okada K, Nannmark U, Vujanovic NL, Watkins S, Basse P, Herberman RB, Whiteside TL. Elimination of established liver metastases by human interleukin 2-activated natural killer cells after locoregional or systemic adoptive transfer. *Cancer Res* 1996; 56: 1599-608.
39. Sandig V, Strauss M. Liver-directed gene transfer and application to therapy. *J Mol Med* 1996; 74: 205-12.
40. Huber BE, Austin EA, Good SS, Knick VC, Tibbels S, Richards CA. In vivo antitumor activity of 5-fluorocytosine on human colorectal carcinoma cells genetically modified to express cytosine deaminase. *Cancer Res* 1993; 53: 4619-26.
41. Guinan EC, Gribben JG, Boussiotis VA, Freeman GJ, Nadler LM. Pivotal role of the B7: CD28 pathway in transplantation tolerance and tumor immunity. *Blood* 1994; 84: 3261-82.

42. Tepper RI, Mulé JJ. Experimental and clinical studies of cytokine gene-modified tumor cells. *Hum Gene Ther* 1994; 5: 153-64.
43. Wilson JM. Molecular medicine - Adenoviruses as gene-delivery vehicles. *N Engl J Med* 1996; 334: 1185-7.
44. Thomas DS, Nauta RJ, Rodgers JE, Popescu GF, Nguyen H, Lee TC, Petrucci PE, Harter KW, Holt RW, Dritschilo A. Intraoperative high-dose rate interstitial irradiation of hepatic metastases from colorectal carcinoma. *Cancer* 1993; 71: 1977-81.
45. Ardalan B, Sridhar KS, Benedetto P, Richman S, Waldman S, Morrell L, Feun L, Savaraj N, Fodor M, Livingstone A. A phase I, II study of high-dose 5-fluorouracil and high-dose leucovorin with low-dose phosphonacetyl-l-aspartic acid in patients with advanced malignancies. *Cancer* 1991; 68: 1242-6.
46. Elias L, Sandoval JM. Interferon effects upon fluorouracil metabolism by HL-60 cells. *Biochem Biophys Res Commun* 1989; 163: 867-74.
47. Houghton JA, Morton CL, Adkins DA, Rahman A. Locus of the interaction among 5-fluorouracil, leucovorin, and interferon-alfa 2 in colon carcinoma cells. *Cancer Res* 1993; 53: 4243-50.

Lynch syndrome (HNPCC): application to the prevention of colorectal cancer

H.J. Järvinen

Second Department of Surgery, University Central Hospital, Helsinki, Finland

Summary

Hereditary nonpolyposis colorectal cancer (HNPCC) is an inherited cancer predisposition syndrome predominantly involving colorectal cancer (CRC), more rarely also endometrial, stomach, ovarian and some other cancers. The clinical « Amsterdam criteria » identify most affected families, but only detection of a mutation in one of the four known DNA mismatch repair genes (MSH2, MLH1, PMS1 or PMS2) verifies the predisposition. The theoretical life-time risk of CRC is 50 % in descendants of an affected parent. In a family with a known mutation, genetic tests can result in either exclusion of increased cancer risk in subjects with no mutation or in increase of the risk to nearly 100 % in mutation carriers. For risk persons colonoscopic surveillance with regular intervals is beneficial enabling removal of adenomas or early detection of CRC. Prophylactic colectomy is another option instead of repeated colonoscopies. Whereas the risk of CRC can be managed reasonably safely, uncertainty remains concerning surveillance of other tumor sites, e.g. endometrial cancer with a life-time risk of 50 %.

Hereditary nonpolyposis colorectal cancer (HNPCC or Lynch syndrome) is characterized by a Mendelian dominant inheritance of cancer predisposition most often involving colorectal cancer (CRC). Special features in CRC are predominance of right-sided tumors, young age of onset and multiple synchronous or metachronous tumors [1]. The other tumor sites associated with the predisposition include endometrium, stomach, ovaries, urinary tract and bile ducts [2, 3]. Clinical diagnosis of the syndrome is difficult, however, and must have support in the family history, *e.g.* as defined by the Amsterdam criteria: (a) colorectal cancer in three or more relatives, one of whom is a first-degree relative of the other two, (b) at least two generations are involved, and (c) at least one of the affected relatives is under 50 years of age when diagnosed [4].

An accurate diagnosis of the predisposition is now possible on the basis of identification of germ-line mutations of one of the four DNA mismatch repair genes *MLH1*, *MSH2*, *PMS1*, or *PMS2* [5-8]. It is not excluded that more genetic loci are involved, but a major part of HNPCC families have been linked with *MLH1* or *MSH2* mutations with about equal proportions [9-10]. Thus far, the genetic diagnosis is relatively complicated and requires first the identification of a specific mutation in each family before predictive genetic tests can be developed and applied in such families. However, in restricted areas, such as Finland, unusually many families share one mutation apparently originating from ancestors in common, facilitating wide application of genetic testing [11].

Preventive measures available *(Table I)*

Lynch syndrome signifies a high risk for colorectal cancer in an identified family. The theoretical life-time risk is 50 % in an at-risk family member, *i.e.* a descendant of an affected parent. This high risk necessitates prophylactic endoscopic screening of unaffected family members according to the model used in familial adenomatous polyposis (FAP) by centralized registries. Endoscopic screening in HNPCC is, however, more demanding than in FAP, because there are no multiple adenomas or other clinical markers antedating the increase of the cancer risk. Thus, whereas periodic sigmoidoscopy is sufficient in FAP to achieve diagnosis in time, full colonoscopy must be performed repeatedly in HNPCC risk members with the aim to remove all polyps from the colon. Furthermore, when increasing age decreases the likelihood of gene carrier status in FAP to nearly nil at 40 years of age if endoscopies are negative, no such age limit can be given in HNPCC.

Genetic predictive testing can intensify the preventive programs when the family members who have not inherited the susceptibility gene defect can be relieved from any increased threat of cancer and omitted from surveillance. On the other hand, this increases the theoretical life-time cancer risk of the true mutation carriers up to 100 %. Quite clearly, knowledge of the mutation status is not without psychological burden for the family members, and the possible untoward effects must be taken in account in the form of individual counceling before applying genetic tests in practice [12, 13].

As a result of genetic test information, the possibilities of preventive measures widen. First, endoscopic surveillance can be targeted for mutation carriers only. Second, the risk of CRC is now so high that prophylactic colectomy arises as a new option which greatly reduces the cancer risk and makes further surveillance of the rectum much easier. A third potentially applicable option is chemoprevention using aspirin, sulindac or some other drugs, or even dietary manipulation, interfering with the development of adenomas or the adenoma carcinoma sequence.

Table I. Preventive measures against CRC in Lynch syndrome.

- Genetic counceling
- Genetic testing
- Repeated colonoscopic screening
- Prophylactic colectomy
- Chemoprevention?

The use of aspirin has already been advocated in the context of various high-risk conditions for CRC [14], but there is not evidence that the effect of aspirin would be similar to that observed after 20 years of regular aspirin use by women under ordinary CRC risk [15]. Serious doubt may be put forward against this idea because the defective DNA mismatch repair function leads to a different tumorigenetic pathway in HNPCC than occurs in most sporadic CRCs [9]. In addition, if the aspirin effect takes tens of years before becoming detectable, the use of the drug should possibly be started soon after birth as the risk of CRC increases already after 20 years of age in HNPCC. At the best, chemoprevention may only decrease the risk for CRC but can hardly totally obviate the need for colonoscopic surveillance.

Colonoscopic screening

The preventive effect of colonoscopy in HNPCC families is based on the presumption that CRC develops from benign adenomas as they do in sporadic CRC [16]. This view is supported by detecting adenomas in 17 to 31 % in HNPCC patients with CRC [17, 18], *i.e.* at least as often as in sporadic CRC [19]. Lanspa *et al.* actually detected more adenomas in 44 HNPCC risk members than in 88 matched controls, 30 *vs* 11 % [20]. On the other hand, Jass *et al.* suggest that adenomas are not more frequent in HNPCC than in the general population but, due to the defective mismatch repair function in HNPCC, the progression of adenomas is accelerated rather than the initiation of the process [21].

Whether more frequent or only more aggressive, adenomas seem to be integral part of the HNPCC syndrome, and therefore, the term « nonpolyposis » is misleading. The explanation for this is the wish to differentiate HNPCC from FAP where the number of adenomas is from one hundred (by definition) to several thousands instead of only a few in HNPCC.

The chief evidence about the benefits of colonoscopic screening in HNPCC comes from the 10-year surveillance study of altogether 251 unaffected family members of 22 HNPCC families [22]. While all the risk subjects were invited for screening, actually only 133 subjects could be enrolled in the program, and the remaining 118 members served as controls. At ten years from the beginning of repeated colonoscopies (or barium enemas) with 3-year intervals, there were six cases of CRC in the screening group compared with 14 in the control group ($p < 0.03$) corresponding to a reduction of CRC rate by 62 %. The effect was ascribed to the removal of adenomas in 22 subjects in the study group compared with only two ($p < 0.001$) in the controls. A further benefit of the screening was the more favorable stage distribution of CRCs detected in screening (all stage A or B) than in the control group (3 stage A, 4 B, 1 C, and 6 D). Correspondingly, none of the CRC patients of the screening group died whereas 5 of 14 (36 %) of control patients died within the study period. No overall survival benefit was demonstrable in our study, but further follow-up has documented two more cases of death in control subjects probably leading to a statistically significant effect even though not formally analysed yet.

The optimal interval between colonoscopies remains controversial. After adenoma removal in normal risk subjects the interval may be safely 3 years or more [23]. However, in a study from the Netherlands, Vasen *et al.* observed 11 « interval cancers » in a screening study of 388 at-risk subjects, meaning that there were no findings in the preceding examination 3 years or less earlier [24]. Three of these cases already had stage C disease, and one further advanced case occurred later [25]. Vasen *et al.* suggest that the screening interval should be 1 to 2 years, at least in gene-tested mutation carriers. On the other hand, very frequent endoscopies cause more inconvenience, anxiety, and they increase the risks of iatrogenic complications. Still some polyps may be missed even by experienced endoscopists. Without serious mistakes in our screening program we have, thus far, maintained the 3-year intervals in the surveillance. We have taken the position that the finding of CRC during surveillance is as such not a failure, and it does not prevent excellent prognosis after surgery in HNPCC patients [26], even though the primary goal is prevention and detection tumors in an adenoma stage. One more point of view is that the family members should not be pressed to come in genetic testing, and irrespective of testing all subjects under risk (50 % or 100 %) should be offered equal preventive programs.

Prophylactic colectomy

The model for prophylactic surgery in a genetically determined CRC predisposition is FAP. It is generally accepted that endoscopic treatment is useless in FAP and surgery is mandatory once the diagnosis is verified by histological demonstration of multiple colonic adenomas, because otherwise CRC develops almost inevitably at the mean age of 40 years. Discussion concerns mostly only whether colectomy and ileorectal anastomosis or restorative proctocolectomy should be used in FAP [27]. The situation is slightly different in HNPCC. First, whereas surgery is undertaken in FAP only when definite clinical disease is already present, in HNPCC the cancer risk is not antedated by multiple adenomas. When one or two polyps are seen in a screening endoscopy, they are usually easily removed by snare, and the remaining colon is « normal » again. Secondly, the actual risk of CRC is not 100 % even in gene-tested mutation carriers of HNPCC family members but lower. The estimated risk was 78 % among 293 putative mutation carriers from Finland [28], and in other studies including 29 and 210 gene carriers the life-time risk has varied from 64 % to 80 % [29, 30]. Thus, 20 to 36 % of the candidates for prophylactic colectomy would probably have unnecessary surgery, even though the surveillance of the remaining rectum would be much easier than total colonoscopies otherwise needed. Third, just like in FAP there will remain a certain risk of rectal stump cancer after ileorectal anastomosis. This residual risk has been estimated to be about 12 % within 10 years after colectomy [31], high enough to necessitate regular endoscopic surveillance.

There are practically no experiences about prophylactic colectomy in asymptomatic mutation carriers of the HNPCC genes. However, it has been demonstrated that CRC is preferably treated by total abdominal colectomy in HNPCC patients due to the high risk of metachronous cancer [32], and there are many examples of cases treated similarly for multiple or large adenomas. Vasen *et al.* made a decision analysis between the options of colectomy and surveillance, and concluded that surgery for a male of 40 years age would give a survival benefit of 8 months over surveillance, and in the case of surgery performed 10 years earlier the increase of life expectancy was 1 to 2 years [29]. Many individual aspects should be considered before applying colectomy for HNPCC gene carriers, such as age, other diseases, compliance with further surveillance, the individual inconvenience or difficulty during previous screenings, and possible previous or present adenomas in the colon. In principle, a life-time risk of 80 % for developing CRC certainly justifies prophylactic colectomy, which can usually be performed with low morbidity and without serious disabling sequelae interfering with normal life [33]. However, when prophylactic colectomy is a necessity in FAP, it must be seen as an alternative option for regular colonoscopic screening in mutation carriers of the HNPCC genes with approximately equal effectiveness until otherwise proven.

Managing with other associated tumors

The progress in the genetic knowledge about the Lynch syndrome has been enormously rapid while the accumulation of proven clinical applications for this information is slow. At present some practical guidelines can be recommended for the prevention and early detection of CRC in HNPCC families, even though the debate about details in screening models certainly continues. There are, however, many other cancer types involved; in fact colorectal cancer covers only about two thirds of the whole tumor spectrum in HNPCC [3]. Preliminary estimates of the life-time risk figures for these other cancers have been presented, such as the analysis of 40 Finnish HNPCC families fulfilling the Amsterdam criteria and being mainly linked with the *MLH1* gene mutations *(Table II)*.

It is interesting that the increased risk for cancer is tissue selective concentrating in some tumor types (see above) but saving other common sites, such as breast, lung, or a number of others [1]. There has been some discussion about possible genotype-phenotype correlation within HNPCC, *i.e.* that the occurrence of the extracolonic cancer may vary according to different mutations in different mismatch repair genes [29]. Such observations are, however, based on relatively restricted series and must be interpreted with caution. At least the division to two types of Lynch syndromes I and II, with or without associated endometrial cancer has little clinical support [3]. If distinct genetic subgroups with different tumor spectra can be documented within the HNPCC entity, this would possibly have influence on the screening protocols. At present it seems that the risk of endometrial cancer is high enough to warrant specific screening programs, but the benefits of such programs still await documentation. It can be anticipated, however, that the impact of the other cancers on the outcome of HNPCC patients will increase in future when the problem of CRC is largely controlled by surveillance or prophylactic surgery.

Table II. Cumulative risks for 6 most common cancer types associated with HNPCC in 40 kindreds (from [28])

Cancer type	Cumulative risk (%)	
	at age 60 years	at age 80 years
CRC	59.1	78.4
Endometrial cancer	35.9	42.6
Gastric cancer	8.8	18.9
Bile tract cancer	5.6	17.5
Urinary tract cancer	2.7	10.2
Ovarian cancer	9.0	9.0

References

1. Marra G, Boland CR. Hereditary nonpolyposis colorectal cancer: the syndrome, the genes, and historical perspectives. *J Natl Cancer Inst* 1995; 87: 1114-25.
2. Watson P, Lynch HT. Extracolonic cancer in hereditary nonpolyposis colorectal cancer. *Cancer* 1993; 71: 677-85.
3. Mecklin JP, Järvinen HJ. Tumor spectrum in cancer family syndrome (hereditary nonpolyposis colorectal carcinoma). *Cancer* 1991; 68: 1109-12.
4. Vasen, HFA, Mecklin JP, Meera Khan P, Lynch HT. The international collaborative study group of hereditary non-polyposis colorectal cancer. *Dis Colon Rectum* 1991; 34: 424-5.
5. Leach FS, Nicolaides NC, Papadopoulos N, Liu B, Jen J, Parsons R, Peltomäki P, Sistonen P, Aaltonen L, Nyström-Lahti M, Guan XY, Zhang J, Meltzer PS, Yu JW, Kao FT, Chen DJ, Cerosaletti KM, Fournier REK, Todd S, Lewis T, Leach RJ, Naylor SL, Weissenbach J, Mecklin JP, Järvinen H, Petersen GM, Hamilton SR, Green J, Jass J, Watson P, Lynch HT, Trent JM, de la Chapelle A, Kinzler KW, Vogelstein B. Mutations of a MutS homolog in hereditary nonpolyposis colorectal cancer. *Cell* 1993; 75: 1215-25.
6. Bronner CE, Baker SM, Morrison PT, Warren G, Smith LG, Lescoe MK, Kane M, Earabino C, Lipford J, Lindblom A, Tannergård P, Bollag RJ, Godwin AR, Ward DC, Nordenskjöld M, Fishel R, Kolodner R, Liskay RM. Mutation in the DNA mismatch repair homologue hMLH1 is associated with hereditary nonpolyposis colon cancer. *Nature* 1994; 368: 258-61.
7. Papadopoulos N, Nicolaides NC, Wei YF, Ruben SM, Carter KC, Rosen CA, Haseltine WA, Fleischmann RD, Fraser CM, Adams MD, Venter JG, Hamilton SR, Petersen GM, Watson P, Lynch HT, Peltomäki P, Meclin JP, de la Chapelle A, Kinzler KW, Vogelstein B. Mutation of a MutL homolog in hereditary colon cancer. *Science* 1994; 263: 1625-9.
8. Nicolaides NC, Papadopoulos N, Liu B, Wei YF, Carter KC, Ruben SM, Rosen CA, Haseltine WA, Fleischmann RD, Fraser CM, Adams MD, Venter JG, Dunlop MG, Hamilton SR, Petersen GM, de la Chapelle A, Vogelstein B, Kinzler K. Mutations of two PMS homologues in hereditary nonpolyposis colon cancer. *Nature* 1994; 371: 75-80.
9. Rhyu MS. Molecular mechanisms underlying hereditary nonpolyposis colorectal carcinoma. *J Natl Cancer Inst* 1996; 88: 240-51.
10. Nyström-Lahti M, Parsons R, Sistonen P, Pylkkänen L, Aaltonen LA, Leach FS, Hamilton SR, Watson P, Bronson E, Fusaro R, Cavalieri J, Lynch J, Lanspa S, Smyrk T, Lynch P, Drouhard T, Kinzler KW, Vogelstein B, Lynch HT, de la Chapelle A. Mismatch repair genes on chromosomes 2p and 3p account for a major share of hereditary nonpolyposis colorectal cancer families evaluable by linkage. *Am J Hum Genet* 1994; 55: 659-65.
11. Nyström-Lahti M, Wu Y, Moisio AL, Hofstra RMW, Osinga J, Mecklin JP, Järvinen HJ, Leisti J, Buys CHCM, de la Chapelle A, Peltomäki P. DNA mismatch repair gene mutations in 55 kindreds with verified or putative hereditary non-polyposis colorectal cancer. *Hum Mol Genet* 1996; 5: 763-9.
12. Petersen GM. Genetic counseling and predictive testing for colorectal cancer risk. *Int J Cancer* 1996; 69: 53-4.
13. Lerman C, Marshall J, Andrain J, Gomez-Caminero A. Genetic testing for colon cancer susceptibility: anticipated reactions of patients and challenges to providers. *Int J Cancer* 1996; 68: 58-61.
14. Marcus AJ. Aspirin as prophylaxis against colorectal cancer. *N Engl J Med* 1995; 333: 656-7.
15. Giovannucci E, Egan KM, Hunter DJ, Stampfer MJ, Colditz GA, Willett WC, Speizer FE. Aspirin and the risk of colorectal cancer in women. *N Engl J Med* 1995; 333: 609-14.
16. Muto T, Bussey HJ, Morson BC. The evolution of cancer of the colon and rectum. *Cancer* 1975; 36: 2251-70.
17. Mecklin JP, Järvinen HJ. Clinical features of colorectal carcinoma in cancer family syndrome. *Dis Colon Rectum* 1986; 29: 160-4
18. Love RR. Adenomas are the precursor lesions for malignant growth in nonpolyposis hereditary carcinoma of the colon and rectum. *Surg Gynecol Obstet* 1986; 162: 8-12.

19. Goligher JC. *Surgery of the anus, rectum and colon*. London: Bailliere-Tindall, 1984, 5th ed: 369.
20. Lanspa SJ, Lynch HT, Smyrk TC, Strayhorn P, Watson P, Lynch JF, Jenkins JX, Appelman HD. Colorectal adenomas in the Lynch syndromes. Results of a colonoscopy screening program. *Gastroenterology* 1990; 98: 1117-22.
21. Jass JR, Cotter DS, Jeevaratnam P, Pokos V, Browett PJ. Pathology of hereditary nonpolyposis colorectal cancer with clinical and molecular genetic correlations. In: Baba S, ed. *New strategies for treatment of hereditary colorectal cancer*. Tokyo: Churchill Livingstone, 1996: 29-39.
22. Järvinen HJ, Mecklin JP, Sistonen P. Screening reduces colorectal cancer rate in families with hereditary nonpolyposis colorectal cancer. *Gastroenterology* 1995; 108: 1405-11.
23. Winawer SJ, O'Brien AG, Ho MN, Gottlieb L, Sternberg SS, Waye JD, Bond J, Schapiro M, Stewart ET, Panish J, Ackroyd F, Kurtz RC, Shike M, and the National Polyp Study Workgroup. Randomized comparison of surveillance intervals after colonoscopic removal of newly diagnosed adenomatous polyps. *N Engl J Med* 1993; 328: 901-6.
24. Vasen HFA, Taal BG, Nagengast FM, Griffoen G, Menko FH, Kleibeuker JH, Offerhaus GJA, Meera Khan P. Hereditary nonpolyposis colorectal cancer: results of long-term surveillance in 50 families. *Eur J Cancer* 1995; 31A: 1145-8.
25. Vasen HFA, Nagengast FM, Meera Khan P. Interval cancers in hereditary nonpolyposis colorectal cancer (Lynch syndrome). *Lancet* 1995; 345: 1183-4.
26. Aarnio M, Mecklin JP, Järvinen HJ. Prognosis of colorectal cancer varies in different high-risk conditions (manuscript submitted).
27. Phillips RKS. Familial adenomatous polyposis: the surgical treatment of the colorectum. *Semin Colon Rectal Surg* 1995; 6: 33-7.
28. Aarnio M, Mecklin JP, Aaltonen LA, Nyström-Lahti M, Järvinen HJ. Life-time risk of different cancers in hereditary non-polyposis colorectal cancer (HNPCC) syndrome. *Int J Cancer* 1995; 64: 430-3.
29. Vasen HFA, Wijnen JTh, Menko FH, Kleibeuker JH, Taal BG, Griffoen G, Nagengast FM, Meijers-Heijboer EH, Bertario L, Varesco L, Bisgaard ML, Mohr J, Fodde R, Meera Khan P. Cancer risk in families with hereditary nonpolyposis colorectal cancer diagnosed by mutation analysis. *Gastroenterology* 1996; 110: 1020-7.
30. Lewis GM, Swensen J, Black J, Burt RW, Skolnick MH, Cannon-Albright LA. Risk of colon and other cancers in an extended HNPCC kindred with a known *hMSH2* gene mutation. *Gastroenterology* 1996; 110: A1133.
31. Rodrigues-Bigas MA, Vasen HFA, Mecklin JP, Myrhoj T, Rozen P, Bertario L, Järvinen HJ, Jass JR, Kunimoto K, Nomizu T, Driscoll DL, and the IGC on HNPCC. Rectal cancer risk in hereditary non-polyposis colorectal cancer after abdominal colectomy. *Ann Surg* 1996; 223: in press.
32. Mecklin JP, Järvinen HJ. Treatment and follow-up strategies in hereditary nonpolyposis colorectal carcinoma. *Dis Colon Rectum* 1993; 36: 927-9.
33. Church JM. Prophylactic colectomy in patients with hereditary nonpolyposis colorectal cancer. *Ann Med* 1996; 28: in press.

Recent advances
in gastrointestinal pharmacology
and therapeutics

Modulation of visceral sensitivity

F. Azpiroz

Digestive System Research Unit, Hospital General Vall d'Hebron, Autonomous University of Barcelona, 08035-Barcelona, Spain

Summary

Physiological stimuli in the gut induce reflex responses that regulate the digestive function. The whole process evolves normally unperceived, but in some circumstances gut stimuli may induce perception. The sensory and reflex responses to gut stimuli are modulated by a variety of mechanisms at different levels of the brain-gut axis. In the first place, the responses depend on the temporo-spatial relationship of the stimuli in the gut; for instance, two stimuli that are well tolerated alone produce discomfort when applied simultaneously. In contrast, somatic stimuli reduce gut perception via *supraspinal mechanisms. The sympathetic nervous system specifically heightens visceral, but not somatic sensitivity. Gut sensitivity is also specifically modulated by cognitive processes such as attention and distraction. Recent data suggest that altered modulation of visceral sensitivity may be the cause of unexplained symptoms in some clinical conditions.*

More than half of the patients in a gastroenterological clinic complain of abdominal symptoms, without any cause demonstrable by conventional diagnostic tests. In the absence of an identifiable organic cause, these clinical conditions are labelled as functional gastrointestinal disorders. Based on the clinical picture, several syndromes have been arbitrarily defined, and the most frequent are noncardiac chest pain, functional dyspepsia and the irritable bowel syndrome. The diagnosis of noncardiac chest pain is applied to patients with thoracic symptoms without cardiac, pulmonary or esophageal disorders. Functional dyspepsia is used for symptoms such as epigastric pressure, fullness and bloating, that presumably originate from the upper gastrointestinal tract and that are frequently precipitated by meals. The irritable bowel syndrome is attributable to the distal gut and is characterized by abdominal pain or discomfort associated to disordered bowel habit. The diagnosis of those syndromes is based on clinical criteria and their underlying pathophysiology is unknown. Some reports during the seventies described sensory disturbances of the gut in patients with the irritable bowel and related syndromes. Ritchie reported in 1973 increased pain from distension of the pelvic colon by inflating a balloon in patients with the irritable bowel syndrome, and this observation was subsequently confirmed by other studies [1]. In 1975, Lasser, Bond and Levitt reported that patients with functional abdominal symptoms complained of pain during intestinal infusion of volumes of gas that were well tolerated by healthy subjects [2]. Unfortunately, this classic observation received at the time little attention and remained anecdotal.

At the beginning of the eighties, the methodology to study the motor function of the gut was fully developed, and in the following years the effort to explain the cause of functional gut disorders was directed towards motility. Motility studies in the eighties described the physiology of gut motor function, that was so far incompletely understood. Furthermore, these studies identified some motor abnormalities of the gastrointestinal tract that caused symptoms. The gastroparesis syndrome was defined as impaired contraction of the stomach and inability to empty its content [3]. Furthermore, the intestinal pseudoobstruction syndrome was defined as chronic or recurrent symptoms of intestinal obstruction without mechanical compromise of the gut, and it was further recognized that the underlying cause was a motor dysfunction of the small intestine due to either a neuropathy or a myopathy [4]. Still, the cause of most functional disorders of the gastrointestinal tract remained unknown. A variety of motility features were described in patients with functional gut disorders, but the relation of these motor patterns to the symptoms was unclear, moreover when the same patterns were also observed in healthy subjects.

In the late eighties it was investigated whether symptoms such as epigastric pressure and fullness after meal ingestion in patients with functional dyspepsia were due to a sort of gastric rigidity, that is, to altered compliance and an abnormal response of the stomach to distension. By distending the stomach, it was observed that the pressure volume relationship, that is compliance, was normal. However, the patients developed their customary symptoms at distending levels that were largely unperceived by healthy subjects [5, 6]. Similar type of gut hypersensitive responses were by then recognized not only in patients with the irritable bowel syndrome [7] but also in patients with noncardiac chest pain [8]. All these data suggested that patients with functional disorders of the gastrointestinal tract might have a sensory dysfunction of the gut, so that physiological stimuli induce symptoms. This idea spread out in the early nineties and prompted the study of visceral sensitivity, that was so far practically unexplored [9].

Responses to gastrointestinal stimuli

Physiological stimuli in the gastrointestinal tract induce specific reflexes to accomplish the digestive function. Normally, the whole process evolves unperceived, and only in some circumstances patients may develop symptoms. Studies on visceral sensitivity in healthy subjects require probing stimuli that induce perception, and this can be achieved using different types of stimulation.

Gastrointestinal distension

The symptomatic response to distension is rather homogeneous from the stomach down to the mid small bowel [10-13]. Most individuals perceive the distensions as a diffuse pressure sensation felt in the epigastrium and the paraumbilical region. A relatively small proportion of distensions in the stomach and proximal duodenum induce nausea, which is rarely induced by jejunal distension. In contrast, jejunal distensions are frequently perceived as colicky or stinging sensation. The intensity of perception is stimulus related, but the same type of sensations are induced by distensions from the threshold for perception up to the threshold for discomfort. Furthermore, the sensitivity along the gastrointestinal tract seems quite uniform, although standardization of distending stimuli in different segments of the gut is problematic. These observations indicate a low discriminative value of gastrointestinal sensitivity, and emphasize the difficulty that exists in ascribing these kind of symptoms (also described by patients with abdominal complaints) to a specific segment of the gut. The distending levels that induce perception and discomfort may vary considerably in different studies depending on several factors, such as the body position, specially for gastric studies, the length of the segment stimulated in the intestine, and the corrections applied. A point of caution in interpreting old studies is the extremely high distending pressures usually reported.

Stimuli such as distension that are not operational in physiological conditions, may nevertheless induce gastrointestinal reflexes. For instance, duodenal distension in dogs elicits a reflex gastric relaxation similar to that induced by nutrients [14]. In a canine experimental model, it was shown that both distension and nutrient effects are mediated by a nonadrenergic, noncholinergic vagal reflex [14, 15]. In humans, duodenal balloon distension also induces gastric relaxation, and the short latency and prompt recovery of the responses suggest that they are neurally mediated [11]. Conceivably, these enterogastric responses in humans are mediated, like in the dog, by a vagal reflex.

Distension of the small intestine also induces intestine inhibitory reflexes. These intestino-intestinal inhibitory reflexes are driven by sympathetic pathways and may relay either at the level of the prevertebral ganglia or the spinal cord [16]. Similar type of inhibitory reflexes in the small intestine can be also elicited by physiological stimuli; for instance, ileal lipids inhibit jejunal activity, a phenomenon called the ileal brake [17]. Conceivably, different reflex pathways may be activated depending on the characteristics and location of the stimuli.

In contrast to the uniformity of perception, the reflex responses to gut distension are quite heterogeneous, and some data indicate that perception and reflex responses are dissociable. Low level distension of the first duodenal portion induces significant gastric relaxation below the threshold for perception. Therefore gastric relaxation is not secondary to perception. Conversely, distension of the proximal jejunum elicits similar perception as duodenal distension, but does not induce significant gastric relaxation. Thus, perception is not dependent on the reflex gastric response [12]. These data suggest that both responses to intestinal distension are induced independently. It is uncertain whether similar conditions prevail at higher levels of distension involving frank pain. Conceivably, nociceptive stimuli could induce gastric relaxatory reflexes [5] and, conversely, a profound gastric relaxatory response could contribute to epigastric discomfort.

Since the enterogastric reflex follows vagal pathways, and perception is mediated by sympathetic-splanchnic afferents, both responses may be produced by different mechanisms. By contrast, both the sensory input and the afferent arm of the intestino-intestinal inhibitory reflex are driven by sympathetic nerves. Short distance anterograde reflexes are released below the perception threshold, suggesting that sensory and reflex pathways are independently activated [13]. These types of unperceived reflexes could participate in the regulation of intestinal capacitance and transit. However, other reflexes, such as the long distance retrograde reflexes, are only activated well above the perception threshold. Hence, these sympathetically-mediated reflexes do not appear to be as dissociable from perception as vagally-mediated reflexes. At this time it cannot be ascertained whether perception and intestinal reflexes share a common afferent path or whether the intestinal stimulus activates two specific systems. Nevertheless it seems that perception and reflex responses may be induced independently. From a pathophysiological standpoint this finding may be very important, because it means that perception and reflex responses to gastrointestinal stimuli may be independently altered in some conditions, and that has been recently shown in patients with functional dyspepsia [18].

Transmucosal electrical nerve stimulation

Testing somatic sensitivity involves a variety of stimuli each activating a specific pathway. For instance, a beta low threshold mechanoreceptors, which produce a faint tactile sensation at levels near the detection threshold, can be assessed by cotton wisps. At detection, electrical stimulation activates the same pathways, but directly stimulating afferent axons independently of the receptors [19]. In analogy to transcutaneous electrical nerve stimulation, transmucosal electrical nerve stimulation can be used as an alternative test of visceral sensitivity. Electrical stimuli have been applied in the esophagus, sigmoid and rectum to study sensory evoked potentials and to induce rectoanal reflexes. In the small intestine, electrical stimulation has been produced *via* intraluminal electrodes. The conductive surfaces of a bipolar electrode are mounted at opposite rims of a suction hole on a tube. When the tube is positioned in the intestine, suction should be applied through the lumen of the tube to ensure firm contact of the electrodes with the gut wall. Transmucosal electrical nerve stimulation is then produced by a constant current stimulator [10].

Transmucosal electrical nerve stimulation of the small intestine induces intensity related perception. The stimulus response curve is similar to that of distension, with a wide span between the intensity to induce perception and that to induce discomfort [10]. Interestingly, more than half of the sensations elicited by electrical stimuli correspond to clinical-type abdominal symptoms such as abdominal pressure, fullness, colicky or stinging sensation, similar to those elicited by distension. Only about one-third of electrical stimuli induce paraesthesia or somatic flutterlike sensation. Conceivably, these sensations originate by stimulation of surrounding somatic structures across the intestinal wall. There is no relation between the intensity of electrical stimulation and the type of sensation elicited, that is, similar sensations are produced by weak, barely perceptible stimuli and by strong uncomfortable stimuli.

Electrical stimuli within a broad range (0.05-1 ms square pulses at 5-100 Hz) elicit similar perception. The intensity of the stimuli to activate sensory pathways and produce perception is more heavily weighted by the duration than by the frequency of the pulses. A 20 fold increase in pulse duration (from 0.05 ms to 1 ms), decreases the intensity of perceived stimuli by a factor of 0.34±0.04; a similar increase in pulse frequency (from 5 Hz to 100 Hz) decreases the intensity by a 0.63±0.07 factor. When the frequency and duration concomitantly increase, the stimulus intensity decreases by the product of both factors (0.22±0.04). Similar type of symptoms are elicited by all stimuli within this range.

Transmucosal electrical nerve stimulation may depolarize all kinds of afferents within the gut wall, including receptors and axons, as well as mechano-sensitive and mechano-insensitive pathways. Hence, whereas distending stimuli activate sensory pathways and induce perception by specific stimulation of mechanoreceptors on the gut wall, transmucosal electrical nerve stimulation induces similar perception by nonspecific stimulation of afferent pathways, that is, without relaying on any specific receptor. Transmucosal nerve stimulation does not modify the intrinsic basal myoelectrical rhythm in the intestine. Furthermore, electrical stimulation induces neither local activation nor reflex inhibition of intestinal motor activity, suggesting that it activates afferent pathways distinct from those activated by distension. This type of electrical stimulation is safe for clinical use because electrical stimuli neither in the jejunum [10, 20] nor even in the esophagus induce changes in cardiac rhythm. Indeed, transesophageal atrial pacing requires considerably longer pulses applied at the closest site to the atrium; pulse shortening or small displacements result in large increments in the stimulus intensity required for atrial excitation.

Thermal stimulation

Nonpainful thermal stimuli provide important information in somatosensory testing. Thinly myelinated A delta fibres mediate sensation of cool, and C-fibres mediate warmth detection. Hence, warmth and cool detection can be used to evaluate these specific pathways [19]. By contrast the responses to visceral thermostimulation remain poorly characterized.

Thermal stimulation of the gut can be produced *via* intraluminal water-filled tubular bags positioned either in the stomach, duodenum or jejunum [21]. The temperature within the bag is continuously monitored by an intrabag telethermometer, and the desired temperature level is achieved by recirculating water at adjusted temperatures through thermally insulated connecting tubes. Temperature changes are achieved fairly rapidly, so that brief stimuli can be tested. The stomach and the intestine exhibit similar stimulus-related thermal sensitivity. About half of the thermal stimuli applied in the stomach (warm and cold alike) are perceived as abdominal pressure, fullness or nausea; the rest of the stimuli induce warm and cold sensation, as corresponded. In contrast, only 10 % of intestinal stimuli induce clinical type symptoms. Gastric stimuli, but not intestinal stimuli, induce changes in gastric tone. Warm stimuli in the stomach induce a gastric relaxation, whereas cold stimuli induce a gastric contraction. The responses have a brief lagtime and revert shortly after discontinuation of the stimulus. Both with warm and cold stimuli the magnitude of the gastric responses is stimulus-related. Thermal sensitivity of the gastrointestinal tract in humans remains poorly explored, and the specific type afferents activated by warm and cold stimuli has not been characterized yet. Nevertheless, thermal stimuli are potentially applicable in conjunction with mechanical and electrical stimuli for the evaluation of gastrointestinal sensory dysfunctions, the same way that differential stimulation refines somatosensory testing.

Mechanisms that determine gut sensory responses

The responses to gut stimuli are determined by a series of factors, and the result depends on their interaction. The responses are unless related, probably due to the discharge rate of the receptors and to the activation of the different pools of afferents (low *versus* high threshold) activated [22]. Furthermore, various mechanisms may modify the sensory input at different levels of the brain gut axis. Conceivably viscero-sensory modulation constitutes an integrated control network, but only a few isolated mechanisms have been so far evidenced.

Muscular activity and compliance of the gut wall

Obviously, the effects of distension depend on the compliance of the gut, and compliance is determined by the muscular activity of the gut wall. Relatively small variations during the cyclic interdigestive motor activity do not affect the responses to distension, but more pronounced changes in compliance do so. Glucagon has a potent relaxatory effect on the gut [13], and markedly increases the compliance of the stomach [23]. Gastric distension at the same pressure levels maintained by the barostat produces larger intragastric volumes and higher perception when the stomach is relaxed by glucagon. However, gastric distension with the same inflation volumes produces higher intragastric pressures and higher perception when the stomach is contracted [23]. Hence, afferent pathways from the stomach convey information about both intragastric pressure and intragastric volume. A simple model of « in series » tension receptors and « in parallel » elongation receptors would explain the gastric responses to distension, but the receptors involved are not fully identified and the actual situation may be more complex. It has been shown that both passive distension and active contraction of the stomach may induce responses in gastric afferents, and these data suggest the presence of muscle tension receptors in the gastric wall [22, 24]. Stretch receptors that respond to distension, but not to active contraction have been also described. This type of stretch receptor probably correspond to the serosal mechanoreceptors described by Morrison, which signal deformation and may thus behave as « in-parallel » receptors. Serosal mechanoreceptors activate spinal pathways, and hence, they may mediate perception [22, 25]. However, it is not clear whether tension receptors may also activate spinal afferents, because in most experiments afferent responses were only recorded in vagal pathways [24].

It has been reported that perception of gastric distension depends on the rate and the pattern of distension. Specifically, perception was more intense with slower rates of ramp inflation, but still higher with rapid intermittent distensions. It was thereby proposed that gastric sensation was induced by activation of different populations of receptors. However, the dynamic effects of distension are difficult to explain, because they are also determined by the visceral displacements within the abdominal cavity at different rates of expansion. Conflicting results have been reported by more recent studies.

The influence of tonic contraction on the response of the stomach to distension provides a basis for understanding the mechanisms by which gastric stimuli may induce symptoms under different conditions. During fasting, the stomach exhibits a tonic contraction. Meal ingestion induces a gastric relaxation, which increases the compliance of the stomach, and hence, the meal is accommodated without increments in intragastric pressure or wall tension. The stomach progressively regains tone during the postcibal period, and this gradual contraction produces gastric emptying [17, 26]. Impaired gastric contraction in the gastroparesis syndrome produces a defective emptying, and these patients may experience symptoms when their hypotonic stomach is over-stretched by food retention. For instance, in these patients with postsurgical gastroparesis, gastric distension with the barostat at relatively low pressures produces a painful elongation of the hypotonic stomach [3].

Conversely, a defective gastric relaxation in the process of meal accommodation may produce increased intragastric pressures and symptoms. There is no direct clinical evidence to substantiate this conclusion, but we have gathered some experimental data in this regard. In a group of healthy subjects we used the barostat to maintain a high intragastric pressure during the postcibal period, simulating a defective gastric accommodation. Increased intragastric pressure induced significant perception of abdominal symptoms, but had only a limited effect on gastric emptying of both solids and liquids [26]. Previous studies in dogs showed that the effect of intragastric pressure on gastric emptying is smaller with nutrient meals than with saline meals. These data indicate that increased intragastric pressure induces symptoms, but also triggers compensatory mechanisms, such as pyloric closure, that modulate the final gastric outflow and maintain the gastric emptying rate of nutrient meals within restrained limits. Gastric distension stimulates gastric secretion, but using a glucose meal we showed that increased intragastric pressure did not stimulate gastric acid secretion, even with high pressure increments that induced discomfort. Hence it seems that the symptoms induced by abnormal increments in intragastric pressure during the postcibal period are not related to increased acid secretion.

Interaction of gut stimuli

Sensory and reflex responses to gut stimuli in humans depend on the temporo-spatial relationship of the stimuli in the gut. The responses to a given stimulus may be modified by either simultaneous or previous stimulation. Perception of simultaneous stimuli is additive, so that the gut responds by a phenomenon of spatial summation; for instance, two distensions that are well tolerated produce discomfort when applied simultaneously. By contrast, the reflex intestinal response increases only to a modest extent [27]. Peterson and Youmans showed in a classic study in the 40's that intestino-intestinal inhibitory reflexes induced by distension in conscious dogs are facilitated by simultaneous distensions, and they coined the term spatial summation [28]. However, these phenomena in humans have more pronounced effects on perception than on intestinal reflexes. Spatial summation can be also elicited by the interaction of different type of stimuli. For instance, low level, just perceived intestinal distension increases perception of transmucosal electrical nerve stimulation applied at an adjacent site. Conversely, low level transmucosal electrical nerve stimulation increases the sensitivity of the intestine to distension, and these effects are not due to changes in muscular activity and compliance of the intestinal wall [20].

The effects of previous stimulation on the responses to intestinal distension are more complex; the effects may be facilitatory or inhibitory depending on the intensity of the previous stimulus and the time interval elapsed from the exposure. Mild distension produces a brief period of local desensitization, and reduces both perception and the reflex relaxation induced by a second stimulus applied 10 seconds later at the same site [27]. However it has been shown that intense, painful distensions may sensitize the sigmoid colon in humans [29]. In fact, intestinal sensitization by previous distension was originally described to enhance intestinal reflexes in dogs [28]. On the other hand, the lack of built-up effects during the stimulation is remarkable; perception of prolonged intestinal distension remains stable at least throughout a 90 minutes period [27]. Both spatial summation and desensitization may be pathophysiologically important, because these phenomena may produce symptoms in response to otherwise well tolerated stimuli, or conversely, may render the gut irresponsive and suppress physiological responses.

Somato-visceral interaction

Following the first enunciation of the gate theory to control somatic pain, it has been shown that a complex neural circuitry, which can be activated by somatic stimuli, is involved in pain modulation. It seems that a neuronal link at the brain stem exerts a descending inhibitory control over spinal transmission, as well as at higher levels of the somatic projection system [30]. Conceivably, spinal and supraspinal circuits with specific modulatory effects can be activated depending on the type of stimulation. Recent data indicate that this modulatory system that reduces somatic nociception also modulates visceral sensitivity. Specifically, it has been shown that application of transcutaneous electrical nerve stimulation on the hand reduces the discomfort produced by gastric and by duodenal distensions. This form of viscerosensory modulation by somatic afferents is exerted without alteration of basal gut tone or visceral reflexes [31]. Some forms of counterirritation or hyperstimulation analgesia require painful stimulation [30]. However visceral discomfort can be reduced by painless somatic stimuli. Furthermore, somatic stimuli may decrease perception of uncomfortable, but not necessarily painful visceral sensations. These observations in humans are supported by experimental studies showing that somatic and visceral sensory input converge onto the same spinal neurons, and that these somatovisceral neurons can be modulated by both segmental and descending inhibitory mechanisms [25]. It has been also shown that noxious cutaneous stimuli in rats inhibit the activity in spinal somatosensory neurons evoked by colorectal distension [29].

The role of these modulatory mechanisms remains speculative. Impairment of a sensory down regulation mechanism could be implicated in the pathogenesis of the visceral hypersensitivity. Furthermore, therapeutic techniques to induce visceral hypalgesia through somatic stimulation could potentially benefit patients with abdominal symptoms. It seems that acupuncture operates by the same type of antinociceptive mechanisms than those activated by other forms of somatic stimulation, and hence, may have similar effects. It has been recently shown that acupuncture increases the tolerance to non-painful gastric distension, and this effect is exerted *via* naloxone-sensitive pathways.

Sympathetic modulation

The sympathetic nervous system regulates gastrointestinal secretory-motor function by a series of reflex arcs, but also participates in the modulation of the sensory responses to gut stimuli. Indeed, it has been shown that several models of experimental stress increase sympathetic activity and modify gastrointestinal responses. However, these methods of sympathetic activation involve cognitive processes or unpleasant somatic sensations, and both factors « per se » may modify visceral perception. Normally, a change in body position from supine to orthostatism induces a sympathetic reflex that increases vascular resistance and prevents a fall in blood pressure. This phenomenon has served as the basis to develop a form of nonhypotensive, nontachycardiac lower body negative pressure, which is a clean and elegant method to produce sympathetic activation without involving pain, stress or changes in basal physiological activity that could interfere with other responses. Using this technique, we have shown that the sympathetic nervous system exerts a modulatory control of visceral but not somatic sensitivity. Increased sympathetic activity significantly heightened perception of intestinal stimuli, but did not modify perception of somatic stimuli [32]. Furthermore, sympathetic activation magnified the relaxatory responses of the gut to both vagal enterogastric and sympathetic intestinointestinal reflexes.

The precise mechanisms by which the sympathetic nervous system modulates visceral perception and reflexes are still unknown. Animal studies have shown that viscerosensory neurons in the spinal cord are controlled by descending excitatory pathways of supraspinal origin. It has been also shown that descending excitatory pathways from suprabulbar areas facilitate spinal sympathetic reflexes, such as the intestino-intestinal relaxatory reflex. Conceivably, sympathetic activation could facilitate vagal reflexes, because the areas of the brain which control preganglionic sympathetic and parasympathetic visceromotor outputs are interconnected. Furthermore, vagal and spinal afferents converge at the brainstem level, and hence, the modulation of spinal afferent input could also affect vagal reflexes.

Alteration of the sympathetic modulation of visceral sensitivity may be clinically relevant. Recent studies have shown that patients with the irritable bowel syndrome display increased sympathetic activity, and precisely these patients exhibit a similar sensory disturbance than that produced by sympathetic activity, namely, they manifest visceral hypersensitivity, but normal or even increased tolerance to somatic stimuli [7, 9, 20, 33].

Mental activity

On top of the modulatory mechanisms stratified at different levels of the brain gut axis, the cortex exerts the final control of visceral perception. In a series of very carefully designed experiments we showed that anticipatory knowledge increases perception of intestinal distension as compared to mental distraction [34]. Furthermore, anticipatory knowledge increases the referral area, and the stimuli were perceived over a wider abdominal region. Mental activity does not modify intestinal compliance or the reflex response to distension. Hence, cognitive processes selectively regulate the sensitivity to gut stimuli, while visceral reflexes operate independently. It is interesting that this type of cortical mechanisms may be activated by hypnosis. It has been shown that hypnotherapy modifies perception of rectal distension in patients with the irritable bowel syndrome without changes in rectal compliance or reflexes. This technique seems a promising tool with potential use in patients with functional disorders of the gastrointestinal tract. Indeed, hypnotherapy has been shown to improve the clinical outcome in patients with the irritable bowel syndrome [35].

Surgical and pharmacological interventions

During the 40's surgical sympathectomy was performed in patients with hypertension for its vasodilatory effects, and it was observed that the patients developed visceral analgesia. In a series of studies it was shown that visceral perception, and specifically gastrointestinal perception, is driven by fibers in the splanchnic nerves and through the thoracolumbar sympathetic chain to the spinal cord [36]. These data are supported by subsequent experimental studies in animals [22, 25]. Although vagotomy has been a very common treatment of duodenal ulcer disease for over 20 years, no evidence supports that the vagus is involved in perception of gastrointestinal stimuli, except for a potential modulatory role [22, 24].

Very little is known about the pharmacological modulation of visceral, and particularly gastrointestinal sensitivity in humans. Some experimental data show that $5HT_3$ antagonists do not modify gastric compliance and perception of distension in healthy subjects. Lysine acetyl salicylate, a cyclo-oxygenase inhibitor, modified neither the normal sensory-reflex response to gastric and duodenal distensions in healthy subjects nor the hypersensitive responses in a group of patients with functional dyspepsia. Interestingly, the peripheral kappa agonist fedotozine has been shown to decrease perception of gastric distension in healthy subjects without modifying compliance. Furthermore, the compound seems effective for the treatment of clinical symptoms in functional dyspepsia [37]. Other compounds, such as somatostatin analogs, [38] and oxytocin [39], have been shown to reduce rectal perception, and conceivably they could also affect the sensitivity of the stomach and small intestine, although it remains unproven. Nevertheless, given the growing interest on gut sensitivity, it is to be expected a flourishment of potential candidates to be tested in the near future. Since the pathophysiology of functional disorders is still incompletely understood [40], it is difficult to design the ideal profile of specific pharmacological agents, but certainly, the availability of nonspecific visceral analgesics would be very useful in the treatment of these patients.

Conclusion

The responses to gut stimuli are modulated by a set of control mechanisms at different levels of the afferent pathways. Altered modulation of visceral sensitivity, either impairment of inhibitory mechanisms or uncontrolled release of excitatory mechanisms, could conceivably result in abnormal exaggeration perception of visceral stimuli. Whether and to what extent these types of sensory disregulations are the cause of the symptoms in patients with functional diseases, is an attractive working hypothesis still to be fully explored.

References

1. Ritchie J. Pain from distension of the pelvic colon by inflating a balloon in the irritable bowel syndrome. *Gut* 1973; 14: 123-32.

2. Lasser RB, Bond JH, Levitt MD. The role of intestinal gas in functional abdominal pain. *N Engl J Med* 1975; 293: 524-7.
3. Azpiroz F, Malagelada JR. Gastric tone measured by an electronic barostat in health and postsurgical gastroparesis. *Gastroenterology* 1987; 92: 934-43.
4. Stanghellini V, Camilleri M, Malagelada JR. Chronic idiopathic intestinal pseudoobstruction: clinical and intestinal manometric findings. *Gut* 1987; 28: 5-12.
5. Mearin F, Cucala M, Azpiroz F, Malagelada JR. The origin of symptoms on the brain gut axis in functional dyspepsia. *Gastroenterology* 1991; 101: 999-1006.
6. Lémann M, Dederding JP, Flourie B, Franchisseur C, Rambaud J, Jian R. Abnormal perception of visceral pain in response to gastric distension in chronic idiopathic dyspepsia. The irritable stomach. *Dig Dis Sci* 1991; 36: 1249-54.
7. Whitehead WE, Engel BT, Schuster MM. Irritable bowel syndrome: physiological and psychological differences between diarrhea-predominant and constipation-predominant patients. *Dig Dis Sci* 1980; 25: 404-13.
8. Richter JE, Bradley LA. The irritable esophagus. In: Mayer EA, Raybould HE, eds. *Pain research and clinical management*, Vol. 9, *Basic and clinical aspects of chronic abdominal pain*. Amsterdam: Elsevier, 1993: 45-54.
9. Mayer EA, Raybould HE. Role of visceral afferent mechanisms in functional bowel disorders. *Gastroenterology* 1990; 99: 1688-704.
10. Accarino AM, Azpiroz F, Malagelada JR. Symptomatic responses to stimulation of sensory pathways in the jejunum. *Am J Physiol* 1992; 263: 673-677.
11. Azpiroz F, Malagelada JR. Perception and reflex relaxation of the stomach in response to gut distention. *Gastroenterology*. 1990; 98: 1193-8.
12. Azpiroz F, Malagelada JR. Isobaric intestinal distension in humans: sensorial relay and reflex gastric relaxation. *Am J Physiol* 1990; 258: 202-7.
13. Rouillon JM, Azpiroz F, Malagelada JR. Reflex changes in intestinal tone: relationship to perception. *Am J Physiol* 1991; 261: 280-6.
14. De Ponti F, Azpiroz F, Malagelada JR. Reflex gastric relaxation in response to distension of the duodenum. *Am J Physiol* 1987; 252: 595-601.
15. Azpiroz F, Malagelada JR. Vagally mediated gastric relaxation induced by intestinal nutrients in the dog. *Am J Physiol* 1986; 251: 727-35.
16. Szurszewski JH. Physiology of mammalian prevertebral ganglia. *Annu Rev Physiol* 1981; 43: 53-68.
17. Malagelada JR, Azpiroz F. Determinants of gastric emptying and transit in the small intestine. In: Schultz SG, Wood JD, Rauner BB, eds. *Handbook of Physiology*. Section 6: *The Gastrointestinal system*. Vol. 1: *Motility and circulation*, 2nd ed, Bethesda MD: *Am Physiol Soc*, 1989: 909-37.
18. Coffin B, Azpiroz F, Guarner F, Malagelada JR. Selective gastric hypersensitivity and reflex hyporeactivity in functional dyspepsia. *Gastroenterology* 1994; 107: 1345-51.
19. Gracely RH. Studies of pain in normal man. In: Wall PD, Melzack R, eds. *Texbook of Pain*, 3rd ed. Edinburgh: Churchill Livingstone, 1994: 315-36.
20. Accarino AM, Azpiroz F, Malagelada JR. Selective dysfunction of mechanosensitive intestinal afferents in the irritable bowel syndrome. *Gastroenterology* 1995; 108: 636-43.
21. Villanova N, Azpiroz F, Malagelada JR. Gut thermosensitivity in humans: sensorial and motor responses. *Gastroenterology* 1991; 100: A505.
22. Sengupta JN, Gebhart GF. Gastrointestinal afferents and sensation. In: Johnson LR, ed. *Physiology of the Gastrointestinal Tract*. Vol. 1, 3rd ed. New York: Raven, 1994: 483-519.
23. Notivol R, Coffin B, Azpiroz F, Mearin F, Serra J, Malagelada JR. Gastric tone determines the sensitivity of the stomach to distension. *Gastroenterology* 1995; 108: 330-6.
24. Grundy D, Scratcherd T. Sensory afferents from the gastrointestinal tract. In: Schultz SG, Wood JD, Rauner BB, eds. *Handbook of Physiology*. Section 6: *The Gastrointestinal system*. Vol. 1: *Motility and circulation*. 2nd ed. Bethesda, MD: *Am Physiol Soc* 1989: 593-620.

25. Cerveró F, Visceral pain: what's in the gut and what's in the brain. In: Taché Y, Wingate D, eds. *Brain-gut interactions*. Boca Raton FL: CRC Press, 1991: 339-46.
26. Moragas G, Azpiroz F, Pavía J, Malagelada JR. Relations among intragastric pressure, postcibal perception and gastric emptying. *Am J Physiol* 1993; 264: 1112-7.
27. Serra J, Azpiroz F, Malagelada JR. Temporo-spatial modulation of perception and reflex responses to intestinal stimuli. *Gastroenterology* 1994; 106: A565.
28. Peterson GC, Youmans WB. The intestino-intestinal inhibitory reflex: threshold variations, sensitization and summation. *Am J Physiol* 1945; 143: 407-12.
29. Ness TJ, Metcalf AM, Gebhart GF. A psychophysiological study in humans using phasic colonic distension as a noxious visceral stimulus. *Pain* 1990; 43: 377-86.
30. Woolf CJ, Thompson JW. Stimulation fibre-induced analgesia: transcutaneous electrical nerve stimulation (TENS) and vibration. In: Wall PD, Melzack R, eds. *Textbook of Pain*, 3rd ed. Edinburgh: Churchill Livingstone, 1994: 1191-208.
31. Coffin B, Azpiroz F, Malagelada JR. Somatic stimulation reduces perception of gut distension. *Gastroenterology* 1994; 107: 1636-42.
32. Iovino P, Azpiroz F, Domingo E, Malagelada JR. The sympathetic nervous system modulates perception and reflex responses to gut distension in humans. *Gastroenterology* 1995; 108: 680-6.
33. Mayer EA, Gebhart GF. Basic and clinical aspects of visceral hyperalgesia. *Gastroenterology* 1994; 107: 271-93.
34. Accarino AM, Azpiroz F, Malagelada JR. Focusing attention at the gut: effects on viscero-visceral reflexes and perception. *Gastroenterology* 1993; 104: A468.
35. Whorwell PJ, Prior A, Faragher EB. Controlled trial of hypotherapy in the treatment of severe refractory irritable bowel syndrome. *Lancet* 1984; 2: 1232-4.
36. Ray BS, Neill CL. Abdominal visceral sensation in man. *Ann Surg* 1947; 126: 709-24.
37. Galmiche JP, de Meynard C, Abitbol JL, Scherrer B, Fraitag B. Effects of fedotozine in chronic idiopathic dyspepsia: a double blind, placebo controlled multicentre study. *Gastroenterology* 1994; 106: A502.
38. Plourde V, Lembo T, Shui Z, Parker J, Mertz H, Taché Y, Sytnik B, Mayer EA. Effects of the somatostatin analogue octreotide on rectal afferent nerves in humans. *Am J Physiol* 1993; 265: G742-5.
39. Louvel D, Delvaux M, Fioramonti J, Bueno L, Frexinos J. Effect of various doses of oxytocin on sensory thresholds in patients with irritable bowel syndrome. *Gastroenterology* 1994; 106: A533.
40. Malagelada JR, Azpiroz F, Mearin F. Gastroduodenal motor function in health and disease. In: Sleisenger MH, JS Fordtran, eds. *Gastrointestinal disease: pathophysiology, diagnosis, management*. Vol. 4, 5th ed. Philadelphia: PA Saunders, 1993: 486-508.

Antidiarrheal therapy

G.J. Krejs

Department of Medicine, Karl-Franzens University, Graz, Austria

Summary

While acute diarrhea is often self-limited and does not need more than general supportive measures and fluid replacement, it is the aim of every physician to find the specific cause of longer-lasting diarrhea and to treat the underlying disease. This may be accomplished by such measures as surgical removal of a VIP-producing tumor, discontinuation of surreptitious laxative ingestion, institution of a gluten-free diet in celiac disease, or immunosuppressives in chronic inflammatory bowel disease. In a number of patients, however, a specific diagnosis cannot be established despite extensive workup and empirical therapy is necessary.

Fluid and salt replacement

When stool volumes exceed one liter per day, dehydration and salt depletion may become prominent. One of the major advances in the treatment of diarrhea came from the observation that the coupled absorption of glucose and sodium in the intestinal villous cell may be unimpaired while secretion occurs at the same time in the crypts of the small-bowel mucosa. Thus, oral administration of sugar-salt solutions may enhance absorption and, despite ongoing secretion, may bring the patient into positive water, sodium and potassium balance. While such oral sugar-electrolyte solutions correct impaired fluid and salt balance, they may not decrease the volume of diarrhea and the patient needs to be forewarned that this therapy may even worsen it. The standard solution that is used for oral fluid replacement is the WHO solution given in *Table I*. Many modifications of this solution have been tested and are used in different parts of the world. It appears that particularly a rice-based oral rehydration solution may be beneficial, since on one hand, starch hydrolysis in many forms of diarrhea is fully maintained by brush-border enzymes and on the other, some of the carbohydrates that enter the colon may be metabolized to short-chain fatty acids. Their absorption stimulates colonic salt and water absorption, and may also salvage some calories.

Table I. Oral fluid and electrolyte replacement

	World Health Organization		Glucose polymer	
	mM	g/l	mM	g/l
Glucose	111	20	–	–
Glucose polymer	–	–	20	20*
NaCl	60	4	120	7
KCl	20	2	10	1
NaHCO$_3$	30	2	0	0
Osmolality (mosm/kg)	331	–	280	0

* Polycose marketed as 47% solution in bottles containing 118 ml; 47 ml of Polycose will contain 20 g of glucose polymer.

In some patients, particularly those with extensive small bowel resection, high sodium concentrations are needed in the oral rehydration solution to achieve a positive sodium and fluid balance. When this is necessary, glucose is best given as a polymer to prevent hypertonicity of the solution. Glucose polymer consists of linear chains of five to nine glucose units and is available as Polycose (Ross Laboratories, Columbus, Ohio) or Moducale (Mead Johnson, Evansville, Indiana), or as Caloreen (Russell Ltd., Wembly Park, England). Glucose polymer is also readily hydrolized in the gut lumen, providing glucose to the sodium glucose carrier in the brush border. Thus, with relatively low osmolality, a high sodium concentration can be provided. The composition of the glucose polymer solution that we use is given in *Table I*. Various flavoring substances can be added to this solution.

Antidiarrheal drugs

Opiates

Opiates have been used for centuries to treat all forms of diarrhea. In chronic secretory diarrhea they remain the first choice for symptomatic therapy. Although opiates show a direct stimulatory effect on intestinal electrolyte absorption *in vitro*, it is probably mainly their antimotility effect that reduces stool volume and frequency in patients with diarrheal diseases. Codeine, diphenoxylate with atropine, and loperamide are most frequently used. Codein and loperamide may be slightly more effective than diphenoxylate. Loperamide has less tendency to cause addiction than codeine and produces less sedation when given in high doses. Codeine, however, is much less expensive. Loperamide also increases anal sphincter pressure and may be of special benefit when fecal incontinence is associated with chronic diarrhea.

Antibiotics

In acute diarrhea, when there is clinical suggestion of infection with a tissue-invasive organism, antibiotics should be given empirically. The antibiotics of choice belong to the quinolone family, *e.g.* norfloxacin and ciprofloxacin. These drugs should be given to a patient who appears to be toxic, has fever, chills and bloody diarrhea. In such cases, antibiotics usually have to be given before a specific diagnosis through stool cultures can be obtained. In patients in whom results of two positive stool cultures are available and the disease has not ceased spontaneously, the agent should be chosen according to sensitivity testing. In most cases this will be ciprofloxacin. While the old literature suggested that the antibiotic treatment of Salmonella infection might promote transition to a carrier state, this does not seem to be the case with the enteritis-type organisms such as *Salmonella enteritidis*. Diarrhea caused by amoebiasis likewise will be treated with antibiotics (metronidazole). For helminthic infections, the appropriate antihelminthic agent will be given.

Other agents

Bismuth

Bismuth salts are poorly absorbed. When present in the lumen, bismuth shows antibacterial activity which probably accounts for its beneficial effect. This has been particularly noted in traveler's diarrhea. Bismuth is mainly available as subsalicylate or subcitrate.

Psyllium

This preparation is mainly used to treat constipation but owing to its capacity to retain water, it is also useful in diarrhea. Stool weight is not reduced but the increased consistency and cessation of watery stool make the diarrhea much more tolerable.

Saccharomyces boulardi

In a number of European countries, various preparations of lyophylized lactobacilli and *E. coli* are available on the market and used quite commonly. Their efficacy has not been proved to this author's knowledge and satisfaction and controlled clinical trials are missing. The yeast *Saccharomyces boulardi* stimulates sodium absorption *in vitro* and has been shown in one clinical trial to prevent antibiotic-associated diarrhea when given concomitantly with an antibiotic. *Saccharomyces boulardi* has not yet been established as a true antidiarrheal agent, *i.e.* one that is effective when diarrhea is first present.

Therapeutic trials

Table II gives a number of agents that are potentially useful in the management of patients with chronic water diarrhea.

Special mention should be made concerning somatostatin since analogs of this peptide are now readily available (octreotide, lanreotide). Somatostatin may specifically decrease the release of a secretagogue from a tumor such as vasoactive intestinal polypeptide in the pancreatic cholera syndrome or serotonin in the malignant carcinoid syndrome.

Gastrointestinal (GI) motility is the extraordinarily complex, highly coordinated neuromuscular process responsible for movement of luminal contents through the digestive system. Smooth muscle cells of the muscularis propria, the final effectors of motility, have innate electrical pacemaker potentials that are under continuous regulation by enteric and extrinsic nerves, circulating peptide hormones, and locally produced chemical mediators. GI symptoms *(Table I)* may result from reduced contractile strength or impaired coordination of contractions in any part of the digestive tract. The precise neurohormonal basis for most disorders has still to be determined.

Table I. Symptoms associated with impaired gastrointestinal motility

Early satiety	Dyspepsia
Loss of appetite	Abdominal distension or bloating
Nausea	Abdominal pain
Excessive eructation	Constipation
Regurgitation	Heartburn
Vomiting	

Drugs affecting GI motility have become valuable in the management of a number of diseases. In particular, newer drugs that possess novel mechanisms of action and that act with greater specificity than the older ones are proving their therapeutic worth. The importance of several recent entries into therapeutics has been twofold: the drugs produce beneficial changes in motility and they have revealed the presence of motility components of disease pathophysiology. As understanding of motility control mechanisms has improved, new uses of established drugs have found application in sometimes unexpected ways. Medications that enhance the transit of material through the GI tract are called prokinetic agents. This class of drugs includes several subclasses each with a distinct mechanism of action. At this time, they are used for their overall benefit on motility. These medications have not been shown to have a selective benefit for a particular motility or symptom complex. Nevertheless, prokinetic agents have been useful in the treatment of a variety of motility disorders.

The potential uses of prokinetic agents are listed in *Table II* [1]. The severity of diseases that may respond to prokinetic agents ranges from the mild constipation associated with irritable bowel syndrome to life-threatening intestinal pseudo-obstruction. In industrialised countries, functional disturbances leading to dyspepsia, indigestion, gastroesophageal reflux or altered bowel habits are extremely common. Together, they generate indirect health care costs second only to those associated with the common cold. Including the over-the-counter component, hundreds of medications have been developed to treat them, at an annual cost in the billions of dollars. Development of new, more effective, prokinetic drugs may reduce patient suffering as well as overall health care costs, but it depends on further clarification of the neurochemical and muscular defects underlying impaired motility. Because many of the patients who would benefit from treatment with prokinetic agents have associated illnesses or are at the ends of the age spectrum, agents with fewer side effects must be sought.

In this paper, the currently available drugs together with their mechanism of action will be reviewed. In addition, the human pharmacology of compounds under current development will be presented.

Table II. Potential uses of prokinetic drugs

Therapeutic uses
    Upper gastrointestinal tract
        Gastroesophageal reflux disease
        Gastroparesis
            Diabetic
            Idiopathic
            Postoperative
        Non-ulcer dyspepsia
        Bile reflux gastritis
        Intestinal manifestations of systemic disorders (*e.g.*, scleroderma, amyloid)
    Small intestine and colon
        Chronic intestinal pseudo-obstruction
        Postoperative ileus
        Irritable bowel syndrome
        Constipation
    Antiemetic
        Hyperemesis gravidarum
        Chemotherapy induced emesis
Diagnostic uses
    Radiographic studies (*e.g.*, small-bowel enemas)
    Aid in intubation of the small intestine (motility catheters, small-intestinal biopsy capsules, suction catheters for bile and pancreatic juice sampling or culture for microorganisms)

How does a drug affect gastrointestinal motility?

Research to determine the specific site(s) of action of prokinetic agents, and the electrophysiologic response of neurons and smooth-muscle cells to them, is an evolving field. Some confusion regarding the cellular mechanisms of action of the prokinetic agents persists as a result of organ- and species specific differences. *Figure 1* shows the different mechanisms through which these agents can influence GI motility [2]. The action of a drug can be due to a specific drug-receptor interaction or can be a direct one on the smooth muscle. The mechanism could also involve a combination of both these effects. An alternative pathway is represented by an interference with the release of one or more mediators affecting GI motility or a central effect. Finally, the precise mechanism of action of an even effective drug could be unknown.

An example of the various sites of action of a drug acting on the cholinergic system at various levels (neurons, nerve endings and thus presynaptic receptors, postsynaptic receptors and acetylcholinesterase) is illustrated in *Figure 2* [3].

Most drugs that affect GI motility do so by means of actions at specific cellular receptors. The receptors may exist physiologically for the purpose of receiving messages from endogenous neurotransmitters, hormones, paracrine and autocrine agents. Most neural and smooth muscle receptors of importance in GI motility occur on the outer side of the cell plasma membrane and penetrate through the membrane to the interior of the cell. Great progress has occurred recently in understanding the structure and functions of membrane receptors. Chemically, receptors that have been characterised consist of complex proteins

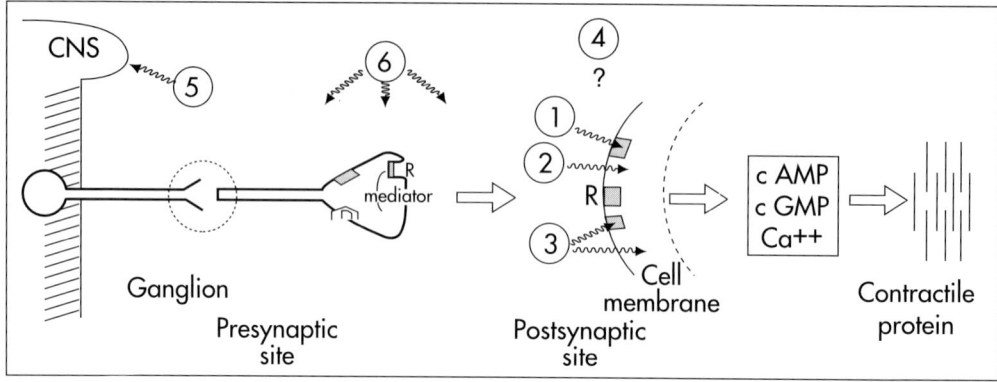

Figure 1. Sites of action of drugs affecting gastrointestinal motility. 1. Specific receptors on smooth muscle cells. 2. Smooth muscle. 3. Receptor and smooth muscle. 4. Unknown site (s). 5. Central nervous system (CNS). 6. Release of mediators affecting gastrointestinal motility (from [5]).

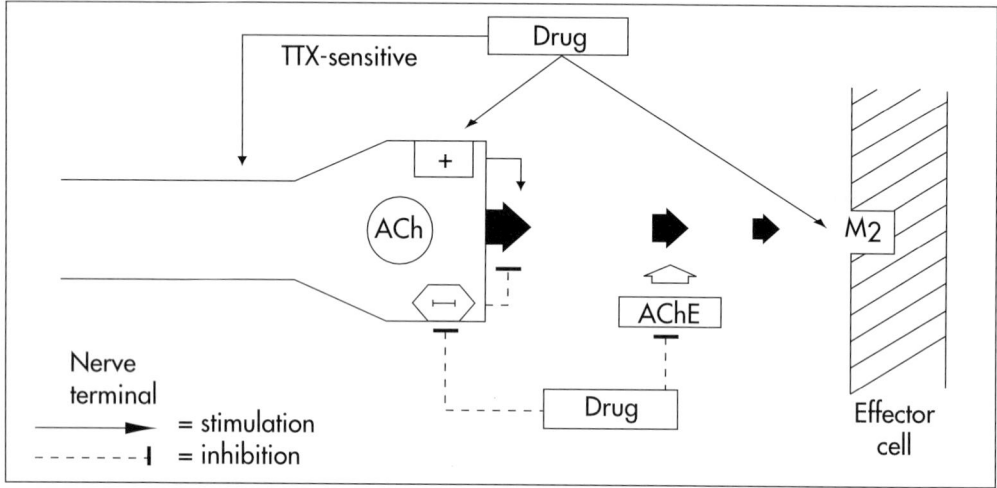

Figure 2. Possible action sites of a prokinetic drug at cholinergic synapsis level. The stimulatory effect can be obtained not only by direct action on the effector cell, but also by stimulation of a pre-synaptic receptor which increases the release of the neurotransmitter (+) or by inhibition of a pre-synaptic receptor which inhibits this release (-), or, lastly, by inhibition of acetylcholinesterase (AchE). Ach = acetylcholine ; M_2 = postsynaptic muscarinic receptor (from [3]).

or glycoproteins. Each receptor consists of three major components: a recognition site, a transduction mechanism, and an amplifier system. The recognition site is that component of the transmembrane receptor that resides on the extracellular surface of the cell and binds to the drug, hormone or neurotransmitter molecules it recognises. The receptor recognition site presents a specific array of physical and chemical features complementary to those of the messenger molecules it binds. There is thus a mutual chemical attraction between the messenger molecule and the corresponding receptor recognition site. Once binding between the drug, hormone or neurotransmitter molecule and the receptor recognition site has occurred, the binding may lead to activation of the transduction mechanisms. It is the ability to activate the transduction mechanism that separates agonists from antagonists. The best characterised of the transducer systems involves proteins that bind guanosine triphosphate (GTP), and the proteins are thus called « G proteins ». The importance of the transducer G proteins is the interesting way they are connected to the amplification system to provide either positive or negative regulatory influences [4].

Three major types of receptor-coupled cellular amplification systems have been identified: ion channels, cyclic nucleotides, and phosphoinositide metabolites. Some receptors, such as the nicotinic cholinergic receptor, are coupled directly to membrane ion channels. Other membrane receptors may be coupled to adenylate cyclase, which generates cyclic adenosine monophosphate (cAMP), or to guanylate cyclase, which generates cyclic guanosine monophosphate (cGMP). Receptors that are positively coupled to adenylate cyclase, such as ß-adrenergic receptors, are linked to a stimulatory G protein (Gs) which is, in turn, linked to the cyclase. Binding of agonist drugs to the ß-adrenergic receptor activates the stimulatory G protein, which increases adenylate cyclase activity. As a result, more adenosine triphosphate (ATP) is converted by the cyclase to cAMP. Through a series of chemical steps, the cAMP results in activation of intracellular protein kinase. Other receptors, such as δ-opioid receptors and some muscarinic cholinergic receptors, may be negatively coupled to adenylate cyclase by means of an inhibitory G protein (Gi). In this case, binding of the agonist to the recognition site activates the inhibitory G protein, which inhibits enzymatic activity of the coupled adenylate cyclase and decreases the amount of cAMP generated. The third major type of amplification system of importance in GI smooth muscle is inositol triphosphate (IP_3). Membrane receptors, such as those for CCK and some muscarinic cholinergic receptors, are coupled through a regulatory G protein to phospholipase C, which mobilises the membrane lipid, phosphatidylinositol 4,5-biphosphate, which is hydrolysed to yield inositol-1,4,5-trisphosphate and diacylglycerol. In terms of contractions of GI smooth muscle, all three types of amplifier systems act to increase or decrease availability of calcium to the contractile proteins [5]. The practical significance of the transducer and amplification systems relies on the potential ability to develop totally new drugs that influence motility by acting on these mechanisms. For example, calcium entry blocking drugs alter motility by decreasing the influx of calcium required by many agents for generation of contractions.

GI smooth muscle cells contain multiple receptors mediating contraction or relaxation. These include receptors to which many physiological substances bind in order to exploit their stimulatory or inhibitory action. From a pharmacological point of view, cholinergic, adrenergic and dopaminergic receptors as well as receptors for serotonin, motilin and CCK are the most important ones since they represent a target of the currently available drugs and compounds under development. An individual cell may of course possess both stimulatory and inhibitory receptors so that the observed action of a drug represents the net effect of excitatory and inhibitory stimuli *(Figure 3)*.

At most neuroeffector junctions, there is normally a balance between the amount of neurotransmitter released from the nerve terminals and the number of membrane receptors in the effector cells. If, for some reason, the amount of neurotransmitter (or a drug that mimics the neurotransmitter) is increased for hours or days, there is often a compensatory decrease in the number of effector cell membrane receptors. If this process occurs acutely

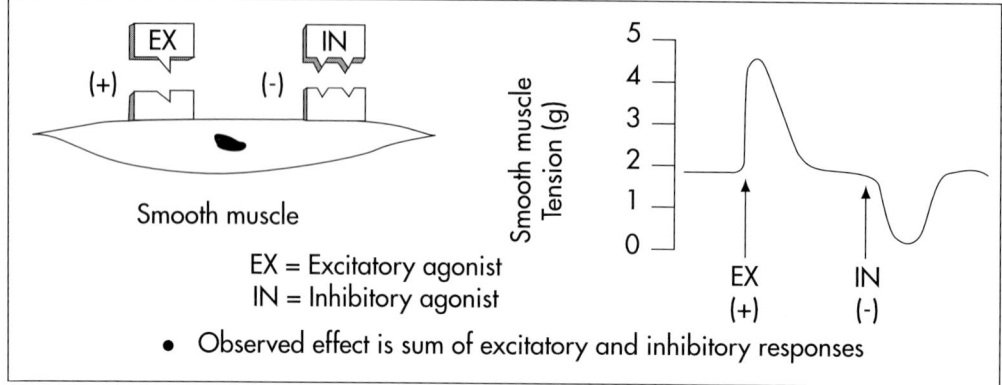

Figure 3. Individual smooth muscle cells possess numerous receptors that recognize many different chemical transmitters and hormones. The individual receptors may mediate either excitatory or inhibitory cellular events. Both excitatory and inhibitory receptors may be located on the same cell, so that a drug action on gastrointestinal motility represents the net effect of both excitatory and inhibitory stimuli (Copyright by AGA®).

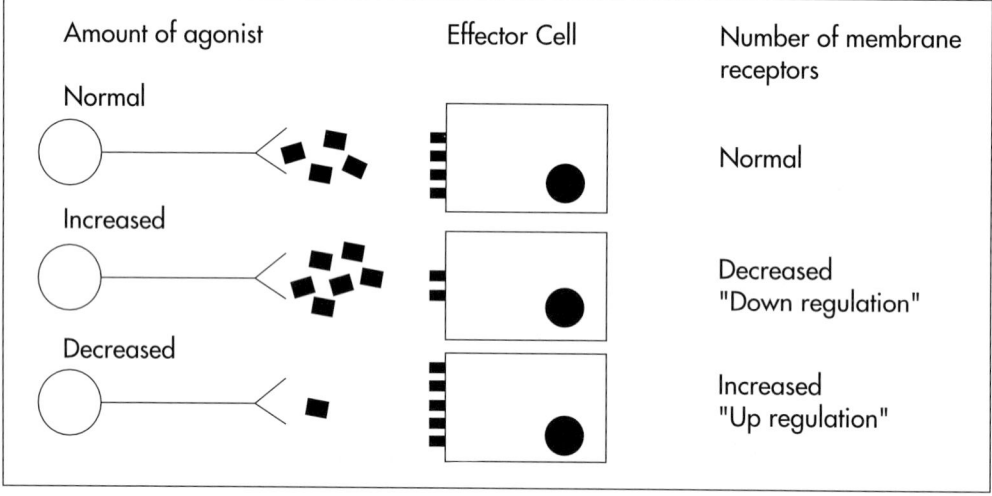

Figure 4. Scheme showing the phenomena of down-regulation or up-regulation that can occur over the time in response to increased or decreased exposure to an agonist (Copyright by AGA®).

(minutes or hours), it is often known as desensitization. If it occurs over longer periods of time, it is often known as down-regulation *(Figure 4)*. In either event, the effector cell becomes less sensitive to the effects of the agonist for the particular receptors. There are many circumstances that result in exposure of effector cells to increased amounts of neurotransmitter or a drug that mimics the agonist actions of the neurotransmitter. For example, long-term treatment with an agonist may result in diminished responses of the effector cells, a form of tolerance associated with down-regulation of receptors. Or a drug may interfere with the catabolism of the neurotransmitter and thereby increase the effective amount of neurotransmitter to which the effector cell receptors are exposed; this also can lead to down-regulation [6].

If, for some reason, the amount of neurotransmitter interacting with effector cell receptors is diminished, there may be a compensatory increase in the number of receptors, termed up-regulation *(Figure 4)*. In this case, the effector cells become more sensitive to the actions of the neurotransmitter. Drugs can produce up-regulation of effector cells by acting presynaptically to reduce the amount of neurotransmitter secreted or by directly antagonizing the effects of the neurotransmitter at effector cell receptors [6].

The phenomena of down-regulation and up-regulation explain many of the changes in sensitivity to drugs encountered in long-term therapy. If the action of the drug is to increase neurotransmission, it may lose efficacy over time because of effector cell down-regulation. If the action of the drug is to decrease neurotransmission, it may lose its efficacy over time due to effector cell up-regulation.

Currently available prokinetic drugs

Schematically, and oversimplicistically of course, one could envisage the motor functions as the expression of a balance at a level of the smooth muscle cells between inhibitory mechanisms mainly regulated by dopamine levels and stimulatory events mainly regulated through release of acetylcholine [7]. It follows from this balance that GI motility can be stimulated both by dopamine antagonists, such as metoclopramide [8, 9], domperidone [10] and L-sulpiride [11], or by substances which release acetylcholine, such as metoclopramide or cisapride [12, 13], or directly by cholinergic drugs which bind and act on muscarinic receptors of the smooth muscle cell, for example bethanechol [7]. A true prokinetic agent is one that not only increases GI motility but also improves the coordination of the various motor functions and accelerates transit through the esophagus, stomach and intestine. *Table III* summarises the differences between bethanechol, which is a motor stimulating compound, and prokinetic drugs like for instance cisapride. Compared to bethanechol, prokinetic agents not only display a stronger action on gastric emptying and peristalsis but also improve antroduodenal coordination.

Table III. Comparison of gastrointestinal motor effects of bethanechol with prokinetics

Effect	Bethanechol	Prokinetics
Muscle tone	+	+
Peristalsis	+	++
Antroduodenal coordination	0	++
Gastric emptying	+	++
Antagonism by antimuscarinics	yes	yes

+ = increase

Amongst the existing prokinetic compounds, dopamine antagonists, on the one hand, and cholinomimetic drugs, on the other hand, should be distinguished *(Table IV)*. Since compounds endowed with dopamine antagonism have the disadvantage of causing neuroendocrine side-effects and/or extrapyramidal dyskinetic reactions (seen especially after metoclopramide), the recently developed non cholinergic non antidopaminergic compound, cisapride, seems to be the most effective one. Its main mechanism of action is considered to be the stimulation of myenteric cholinergic nerves with consequent increase of acetylcholine release [12, 13].

Table IV. Currently available motor stimulating compounds

Mechanism of action	Compound
Direct action on muscarinic receptors	Bethanechol
	Metoclopramide
Dopamine-receptor (D_2) antagonism	Metoclopramide
	Clebopride
	L-sulpiride
	Domperidone
Enhanced acetylcholine release	Metoclopramide
	Cisapride
Interaction with serotonin receptors (5-HT_3 antagonism*/5-HT_4 agonism)	Cisapride

* Metoclopramide also displays 5-HT_3 antagonist activity at very high doses (as those used to prevent chemotherapy induced emesis).

The mechanism by which cisapride and other substituted benzamides (*e.g.* zacopride, renzapride and mosapride) cause the release of acetylcholine is controversial. Early studies indicated that cisapride prokinetic effect might be mediated *via* antagonism of 5-hydroxytryptamine (5-HT; serotonin) type 3 receptors [14]. This hypothesis is inconsistent with the lack of prokinetic effects of other known 5-HT_3 antagonists. Ondansetron, a selective 5-HT_3 receptor antagonist, has been actually shown to decrease colonic motility [15]. Boeckxstaens *et al.* [16] demonstrated that stimulation of neuronal 5-HT_3 receptors in dog terminal ileum and ileocolonic junction results in the release of an inhibitory nonadrenergic noncholinergic neurotransmitter, causing relaxation.

In addition to their antagonist effect on 5-HT_3 receptor, substituted benzamides also stimulate a subpopulation of serotonin receptors, the 5-HT_4-receptors [16]. Schuurkes *et al.* [17] have shown the effects of cisapride to be mediated by these receptors in guinea pig ileum and colon. Cisapride was found able to potentiate fast nicotinic excitatory postsynaptic potentials in S-type enteric neurons of the guinea pig ileum, an effect that is antagonized by low concentrations of tropisetron (ICS 205-930), which blocks 5-HT_4 receptors, but not by the 5-HT_3 receptor antagonist ondansetron [17,18].

The possibility that cisapride may influence the transmission of other intrinsic chemical messengers has also been examined. Tari *et al.* [19] found that cisapride increases tissue concentrations of ß-endorphin at several sites and decreases the concentration of substance P in the muscle layers of the rectosigmoid colon. In the fasting state, cisapride induces a release of PP *via* cholinergic and probably vagal mechanisms, and a release of motilin most likely secondary to increased mechanical activity [20]. It is unclear how PP could contribute to cisapride effects, but motilin may amplify its motor stimulating properties.

The post-prandial release of motilin is less documented, but – if present – could contribute to the acceleration of gastric emptying seen after cisapride.

Cisapride stimulates antroduodenal motility by enhancing the amplitude of antral contractions and by enhancing antroduodenal coordination *(Figure 5)*, an effect which has been reported also for metoclopramide and domperidone [21].

Compared with metoclopramide and domperidone, cisapride (and some new agents under development) displays not only a different drug-receptor interaction profile *(Table V)* but also a different activity pattern. Indeed, although all the gastrokinetic drugs affect upper GI motility, only the more recent ones display an activity on the lower gut. Also the safety profile of these compounds changed over the time, the more recent compounds being almost devoid of untoward effects *(Table VI)*.

The main pharmacokinetic parameters of the currently available prokinetic agents are summarized in *Table VII* [22]. Usually, metoclopramide and domperidone are given in

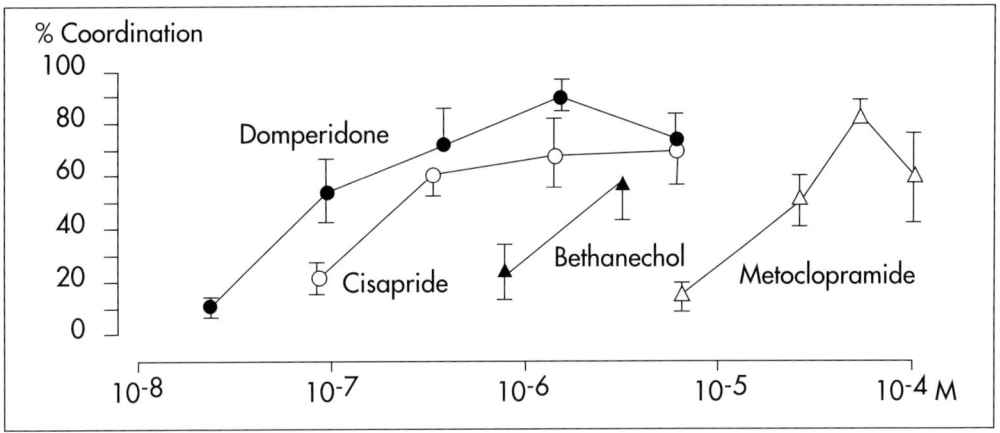

Figure 5. Dose-response of antroduodenal coordination to several prokinetic agents. Improved coordination is reflected by increased transmission of antral contractions to the duodenal segment of a guinea pig gastroduodenal preparation *in vitro* (from [21]).

Table V. Prokinetic compounds: drug-receptor interaction

Compound	D_2 receptor antagonism	5-HT$_3$ receptor antagonism	5-HT$_4$ receptor agonism	Motilin receptor agonism	CCK-A receptor antagonism
Metoclopramide	Yes	Yes	No	No	No
Domperidone	Yes	No	No	No	No
Cisapride	No	Yes	Yes	No	No
Erythromycin	No	No	No	Yes	No
Loxiglumide	No	No	No	No	Yes

Table VI. Prokinetic compounds: comparison of activity profiles

Compound	Crossing BB barrier	Antiemetic effect	Activity on proximal gut	Activity on distal gut	Untoward effects
Metoclopramide	Yes	Yes	Yes	No	Many
Domperidone	No	Yes	Yes	No	Some
Cisapride	No	No	Yes	Yes	Few
Erythromycin	No	No	Yes	Yes	Few
Loxiglumide	Yes	No	Yes	Yes	Few

Table VII. Pharmacokinetic parameters of the currently available prokinetic compounds (modified from [22]

Drug	Adult dose (mg)	Pediatric dose (mg/kg)	T_{max} (h)	Half-life (h)	Bio-availability (%)	Excretion
Cisapride	5-20 tid	0.2 tid-qid	2	7-15	40-50	urine, stool
Metoclopramide	10 qid	0.1 qid	1	2.6-5.2	32-97	urine
Domperidone	10 qid	0.6 qid	0.5-1	7.5	12-18	urine, stool

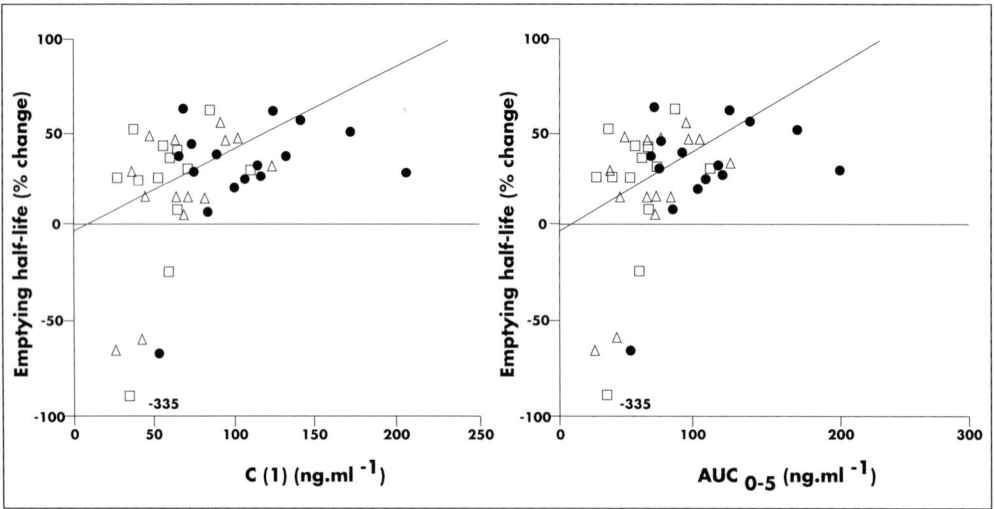

Figure 6. Relation between the improvement in gastric emptying half-times [100-(% $t_{1/2}$ changes vs basal $t_{1/2}$)] and: **a)** cisapride plasma concentrations 1 h after the lunch-time dose [C(1)] (r = 0.33; p < 0.05); **b)** the areas under plasma concentration-time curves from the sample before the lunchtime dose to that 5 h later (AUC_{0-5}) (r = 0.38; p < 0.01). □ cisapride 10 mg 30 min before breakfast and placebo before lunch (1 × 10 mg); △ cisapride 20 mg 30 min before breakfast and placebo before lunch (1 × 20 mg); • cisapride 10 mg 30 min before breakfast and before lunch (2 × 10 mg) (from [23]).

3-4 daily doses before meals, based on the rationale that peak plasma concentrations would occur at the appropriate times to accelerate gastric emptying. However, since cisapride has an elimination half-life which is significantly longer than those of the former drugs, a twice daily regimen is effective. In patients with idiopathic gastroparesis, Corinaldesi et al. [23] were able to show a significant correlation between cisapride plasma concentration and changes in gastric emptying *(Figure 6)*. Peak concentrations of cisapride greater than 60 ng/ml were invariably associated with acceleration in emptying rate.

The existence of a threshold plasma concentration below which cisapride would have less of a prokinetic effect could – at least partially – account for some discrepancies concerning the drug effects found in the literature. Since acceleration of gastric emptying is related to cisapride plasma concentration, non-responders should be studied in depth and treatment with higher doses be explored.

Future prokinetic compounds

Although GI motility has been yet stimulated through the use of dopamine antagonists or of direct or indirect cholinergic drugs, recent evidence strongly suggests that blockade of CCK-receptors and stimulation of motilin receptors are also promising avenues. Since drugs acting on 5-HT receptors, like cisapride, are presently the best available motor stimulating compounds, new derivatives are being developed as gastrokinetic drugs.

CCK receptor antagonists

It is well known that minute amounts of CCK are able to affect GI motility under all the possible *in vivo* and *in vitro* experimental conditions in both animals and humans [24], thus suggesting this action on the gut to be one of the physiological actions of the peptide. A summary of CCK effects on human GI motility is showed in *Table VIII* [24-26]. CCK was found to reduce lower esophageal sphincter pressure (LESP) in a dose-dependent manner [27] and to partially inhibit the stimulatory effect of pentagastrin. The fat-induced inhibition of LES pressure is probably related to CCK release from the duodenum. A recent investigation [28] also showed an increase of post-prandial transient LES relaxations (TLESRs) after endogenous CCK (released by high fat meal). Gastric emptying of both liquids and solids is significantly delayed by CCK and its synthetic derivatives (like for instance CCK-OP and the amphibian peptide caerulein) [29]. The mechanism through which CCK inhibits gastric emptying probably involves a drop in intragastric pressure due to relaxation of the proximal stomach together with a contraction of the antropyloric region, where the peptide decreases the motility index and the basal frequency of the electric rhythm. As far as the small and large intestine are concerned, CCK has a mixture of stimulatory and inhibitory effects on gut motility, although the stimulatory ones are largely predominant. In the first part of the duodenum, the peptide has an inhibitory effect on the motility index and basic electric rhythm (BER) frequency, which resembles its relaxant effect on the sphincter of Oddi.

It is now well established that CCK exerts its physiological effects through binding with specific receptors located on target cells. At least two different receptors mediate CCK biological actions: CCK-A and CCK-B receptors [30, 31]. The CCK-A receptor mediates most of the activities of CCK in the GI system. It is present on the pancreatic acinar cells, gallbladder as well as alimentary tract muscle, neurones in the myenteric plexus, vagal afferents from the GI tract and also in certain brain nuclei. The CCK-B receptor is mainly a brain receptor and probably modulates the actions of CCK in the central nervous system (CNS). It is worth mentioning that the gastrin receptor is similar to the CCK-B receptor [32] and, to date, no compounds have been described that clearly distinguish between these two receptors.

Table VIII. Effects of CCK on human digestive motility

- Dose-dependent reduction of LESP
- Inhibition of pentagastrin-induced increase of LESP
- Relaxation of the proximal stomach and contraction of the antropyloric region
- Inhibition of gastric emptying of both solids and liquids
- Inhibition of mechanical and electrical activity of the duodenum
- Stimulation of small bowel and colonic motility

Eight classes of CCK-antagonists including hundreds of compounds have been described [30, 31]. These antagonists have been used successfully in animals to confirm the classical actions of CCK as well as to explore novel activities including its role as a neuropeptide. Amongst the compounds characterised as selective CCK-A receptor antagonists, two molecules have reached clinical trials, namely devazepide and loxiglumide. Since the former was discontinued during early clinical development, almost all the clinical investigations have been performed with loxiglumide.

Effect of loxiglumide on human digestive motility

Katschinski et al. [33] studied the effect of loxiglumide on esophageal motility in healthy volunteers. The compound was administered intravenously (10 mg.kg^{-1}.h^{-1}) in basal conditions and during an intraduodenal infusion of a Lundh test meal. Loxiglumide only slightly affected esophageal peristalsis in the interdigestive state *(Table IX)* and had no effect in the post-prandial period. No effect on basal LESP was evident, but the compound was able to counterbalance the meal-induced decrease in sphincter pressure. Provided this action of loxiglumide be confirmed also in patients with GERD, the drug could be useful to prevent or reduce post-prandial reflux.

Table IX. Effect of loxiglumide (10 km/kg/h) on interdigestive esophageal motility in healthy volunteers (from [33])

Parameter	Saline	Loxiglumide	Significance
LESP (mmHg)	24.9 ± 2.9	27.2 ± 2.7	NS
Motility index (mmHg x s)	188.1 ± 22.6	210.8 ± 29.5	p < 0.05
Duration of contraction	3.6 ± 0.1	3.9 ± 0.2	p = 0.06
Peristaltic velocity (cm/s)	3.2 ± 0.2	2.8 ± 0.1	p = 0.01

NS = not significant

Bearing in mind the inhibitory effect of CCK on gastroduodenal motility, one could predict that CCK-A receptor blockade alone would result in an acceleration of emptying rate. This prokinetic activity of CCK-A antagonists is rarely observed however, at least in the experimental animals. In fact, while CCK-A receptor antagonists constantly block CCK-induced inhibition of gastric motility [29], their effect on basal gastric emptying is variable and strictly depends on the experimental conditions. Amongst these, the nature (solid or liquid) and composition of the test meal seem to be the most important ones [34-36].

Results from human studies are in line with those obtained in experimental animals *(Table X)*. The effect of loxiglumide on gastric emptying in man was first evaluated by means of radioopaque markers ingested with three different meals [37]. Although loxiglumide significantly accelerated the emptying of the markers after a liquid test meal, no effect was evident when they were ingested with the guar or glucose meals. These apparent contrasting effects can be easily explained taking into account that only the mixed meal releases endogenous CCK and shows that loxiglumide has no intrinsic effect on gastric emptying. However, Fried *et al.* [38] were able to evidence with this CCK-A antagonist an acceleration of emptying rate (evaluated by gamma scintigraphy) not only of a mixed liquid meal (Ensure®) but also of a glucose meal. Besides the different techniques of gastric emptying measurement (radiography *versus* scintigraphy), the different glucose concentrations (5 % *versus* 20 %) and caloric contents (100 kcal *versus* 400 kcal) of the two glucose meals as well as the dose (30 mg/kg *versus* 10 mg/kg/h) and route of administration (oral *versus* intravenous) of loxiglumide may help to explain discrepancies in findings. It is worth mentioning that Corazziari *et al.* [39], by using another technique (ultrasonographic measurement of the antral volume) and a solid meal, were unable to confirm the gastrokinetic effect of loxiglumide. On the other hand, in one study [40], devazepide (10 mg orally) proved to be unable to modify gastric emptying of either solids and liquids whereas in another investigation [41] the same dose was found capable of significantly accelerating the early emptying rate of a liquid mixed meal.

Table X. Effect of the CCK-A antagonists, released for human studies, on basal gastric emptying in healthy subjects

Authors	Ref.	Type of meal	Antagonist	Dose (mg/kg)	Route of administration	Effect
Meyer et al.	37	Guar liquid meal	Loxiglumide	30 mg/kg	oral	0
		5% glucose solution	Loxiglumide	30 mg/kg	oral	0
		Mixed liquid meal	Loxiglumide	30 mg/kg	oral	+
Fried et al.	38	20% glucose solution	Loxiglumide	10 mg/kg	i.v.	+
		Mixed liquid meal	Loxiglumide	10 mg/kg	i.v.	+
Corazziari et al.	39	Mixed solid meal	Loxiglumide	800 mg	oral	0
Liddle et al.	40	Mixed solid/liquid meal	Devazepide	10 mg	oral	0
Cantor et al.	41	Mixed liquid meal	Devazepide	10 mg	oral	+[a]

i.v. = intravenously; + acceleration of emptying rate; 0 = no effect on emptying rate; [a]acceleration evident only in the early of the emptying process (*i.e.* the first 75 min).

The effects of loxiglumide on small bowel transit time and colonic transit time were studied in healthy volunteers by means of the H_2 breath test and radiopaque markers, respectively [37]. In experiments, where intestinal transit was evaluated, the CCK-antagonist was infused intravenously (10 $mg.kg^{-1}.h^{-1}$) starting 60 minutes before intraduodenal administration of the test meal whereas, in those concerning colonic transit, the administration of erythromycin stearate (1 g) and erythromycin acistrate (2'-acetyl-erythromycin stearate) (0.8 g) shortens the oro-caecal transit time (as measured by hydrogen breath test) in healthy volunteers [77]. Some subjects experienced adverse GI untoward effects with erythromycin stearate compared with none of the erythromycin acistrate group.

Little attention has been paid to a possible role for motilin in the regulation of motility in the large intestine. It was reported that the peptide increases colonic myoelectric activity and pressures as well as initiates a premature giant MMC in the caecum of the dog [48]. These effects have however been considered pharmacologic rather than physiological ones. The recent discovery of motilin receptors in colonic smooth muscle [78], with a density higher than that found in the antrum and duodenum, shed new light on the physiological role of motilin and opened new perspectives for the therapeutic applications of macrolides with motilin agonist properties.

In isolated colonic smooth muscle [79], erythromycin displaced ^{125}I-labeled motilin, thus suggesting the two substances to bind the same receptors. When whole colonic transit, evaluated by means of radioopaque markers, was studied in healthy volunteers given erythromycin (250 mg orally q.i.d. for 8 days), it was accelerated (although not significantly) by the drug. There was, however, a significant decrease in transit time of the right colon, thus suggesting a shift in fecal distribution [79]. Bassotti *et al.* [80], however, found a significant increase of segmental contractile activity in the sigmoid, but not transverse and descending colon of chronically constipated subjects given intravenous erythromycin (500 mg.h^{-1}). Taken together, these data suggest that this macrolide antibiotic could be helpful in the treatment of constipation.

One investigation [81] attempted to find a benefit with erythromycin in treating postoperative ileus but preliminary results were not encouraging. However, appearance of flatus or bowel movements were taken as valuable parameters in this trial and a recent study [82] has shown that the postoperative motor complex do not correlate in time with first passage of flatus or stool. Therefore, a different end point (*i.e.* the return of IMC) should be chosen when investigating the clinical usefulness of macrolide antibiotics on postoperative ileus.

Although erythromycin induces stimulation of phase III activity in the upper gut of patients (both adults and children) with small bowel hypomotility due to chronic pseudo-obstruction [83], clinical evidence of benefit is lacking.

Development of motilinomimetics

While screening a number of erythromycin derivatives, Omura *et al.* [84] discovered a group of compounds with a loss in antibiotic potency, but an increased potency to induce contractions and to mimic motilin. For this reason Itoh and Omura [85] proposed to give the name motilides to all macrolides with a) a direct contractile effect *in vitro* on rabbit duodenal segments; b) the capacity to induce *in vivo* phase III activity in dogs.

In a detailed study of 73 macrolide derivatives [86], the potency to displace motilin bound to its receptor was well correlated to the potency in the tissue bath. Therefore binding to the rabbit smooth muscle motilin receptor can be considered a good model for the development of motilides [87]. Peeters [87] proposed to use the name motilinomimetics for any compound able to interact with the motilin receptor, because the discovery of the prokinetic properties has also stimulated a renewed interest into motilin. Motilinomimetics may therefore in the future consist of two classes of compounds: motilides (macrolide derivatives) and motilin analogs.

Table XI shows a list of motilinomimetics that have been synthesized so far, for most of which the interaction with motilin receptors has been determined [88-96]. Further development will depend on the lack of antimicrobial activity and the absence of fading of the prokinetic effect during prolonged administration.

Table XI. Motilinomimetics under development

Authors	Year	Ref.	Compound	Company	Structural features[1]	pK_{d}[2]
Depoortere et al.	1990	88	EM-523	Takeda, Japan	14; enol	8.40
Sakai et al.	1993	89	EM-574	Takeda, Japan	14; enol	7.94
Hanyu et al.	1993	90	KW-5139	Kyowa, Japan	[Leu[13]]-po-motilin	9.18
Nellans et al.	1994	91	A-81229	Abbott, USA	14; enol	8.14
Takanashi et al.	1994	92	GM-611	Chugai, Japan	14; enol	8.38
Greenwood et al.	1994	93	LY-267108	Lilly, USA	12; enol	ND
Eeckhout et al.	1994	94	KC-11458	Solvey, Germany	12; enol	ND
Macielag et al.	1995	95	OHM-11638	Ohmeda, USA	Motilin fragment analogue	8.94
Maes et al.	1996	96	ABT-229	Abbott, USA	12; enol	ND

[1] Number of atoms in the macrolide ring; presence of the enol configuration
[2] Negative logarithm of the dissociation constant for the motilin receptor
ND = not determined

Drugs acting on 5-HT receptors

The use of selective agonists and antagonists allowed to establish that the biological actions of 5-hydroxytryptamine (5-HT) are mediated by at least 4 types of receptors: $5-HT_1$-like, $5-HT_2$, $5-HT_3$ and the recently described $5-HT_4$ receptor [97]. It is well known that metoclopramide is an effective, albeit weak, antagonist of $5-HT_3$ receptors which have been found only associated with peripheral autonomic, afferent and enteric neurons [98]. The effectiveness – as antiemetic and motor stimulating compounds – of some selective $5-HT_3$ antagonists (like for instance ondansetron, granisetron and tropisetron), devoid of any effect at dopamine receptors, suggested that blockade of these sites plays an important role in the mechanism of action of metoclopramide [99]. As a consequence, the potential of $5-HT_3$ antagonists as gastrokinetic drugs has been explored in both animals and humans.

Animal experiments have shown that almost all the available $5-HT_3$ antagonists (namely ondansetron, granisetron, tropisetron, alosetron and cilansetron) are capable of accelerating gastric emptying of either nutrient and non-nutrient meals [100]. In humans, gastric emptying of both solids and liquids is accelerated by intravenous [101] and oral [102] administration of tropisetron, an effect not found in patients with anorexia nervosa [103]. On the other hand, ondansetron proved to be unable to modify emptying rate in healthy volunteers [104, 105] or in patients with persistent nausea [106].

The effect of tropisetron on esophageal motility was studied in healthy volunteers by Stacher et al. [107], who reported a significant and long-lasting increase of LESP after intravenous administration of the compound (20 mg), an effect not seen after oral administration [108].

5-HT_3-receptor antagonists delay orocecal and colonic transit times [15, 105] and also reduce the tonic gastrocolic response to feeding [109, 110]. In patients with carcinoid diarrhea, a 5-HT_3-antagonist proved to be capable of correcting the hypertonic colonic response to food [111]. These data provide the rationale for ongoing trials with these drugs in (diarrhea-predominant) irritable bowel syndrome (IBS).

Table XII. The most investigated drugs acting on 5-HT receptors, some of which are presently under development

Authors	Year	Ref.	Compound	Company	5-HT_4 agonism	5-HT_3 antagonism	D_2 antagonism
Sanger	1987	112	Renzapride	Smithkline Beecham, UK	yes	yes	no
Yoshida et al.	1989	113	Mosapride	Astra, Sweden	yes	yes	no
Fernandez et al.	1990	114	Pancopride	Almirall, Spain	yes	yes	no
Turconi et al.	1991	115	BIMU 1	Boehringer Ingelheim, Germany	yes	yes	no
Gullikson et al.	1992	116	Zacopride	Synthelabo, France	yes	yes	no
Flynn et al.	1992	117	SC-53116	Searle, USA	yes	yes	no
Clark et al.	1993	118	RS-56532	Hokuriku Seiyaku, Japan	yes	yes	no
Buchheit et al.	1995	119	SDZ-HTF-919	Sandoz, Switzerland	yes*	yes	no

* Potent but partial agonist

The lack of correlation between the potency of these compounds as 5-HT_3 receptor antagonists and their ability to stimulate GI motility suggests that mechanisms other than blockade of 5-HT_3 receptors should be involved in their motor stimulating activity [62]. Rather, an agonistic activity at level of 5-HT_4 receptors, located on nerve terminals of both cholinergic interneurons and motor neurons and whose stimulation increases acetylcholine release, seems to be the key mechanism of established (e.g. cisapride) and new (Table XII, [112-119]) prokinetic compounds [97, 120, 121]. The matter is rather puzzling since some 5-HT_3 antagonists display agonistic properties at level of 5-HT_4 receptors, some are devoid of such an effect while tropisetron (ICS 205-930) actually behaves (at high doses) as a 5-HT4 antagonist (Figure 7, [97]). Whatever the receptor subtype involved, drugs acting on 5-HT receptors are capable of affecting upper and lower GI motility and, provided their action be confirmed in patients, new prokinetic compounds belonging to this class of drugs will be soon available for clinical use.

Hormonal peptides

Octreotide

Native somatostatin has variable effects on motor activity of the GI tract depending on the physiological state and region studied. In the stomach, somatostatin inhibits the normal

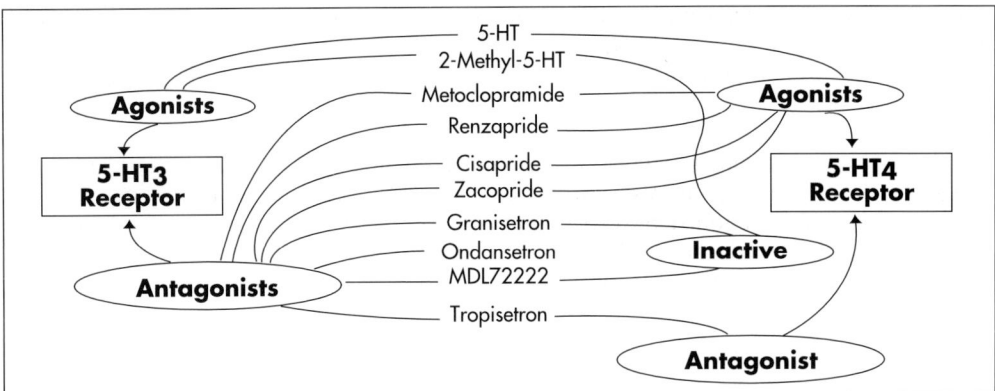

Figure 7. Activity of some motor stimulating compounds at 5-HT$_3$ and 5-HT$_4$ receptor level (from [97]).

occurrence of cyclic interdigestive and fed motor activities [122]. In the intestine, the peptide initiates ectopic fronts under basal conditions but inhibits fed motility [123].

In healthy subjects, somatostatin initiates a propagative pattern of motor stimulants in the duodenum, with a shortened cycle length of 40 min [124]. The long-acting somatostatin analog, octreotide [125], evokes a similar intestinal pattern of contractions in dogs [126]. When given (50 µ/day subcutaneously) to patients with scleroderma and intestinal pseudo-obstruction [127], octreotide proved to be an effective prokinetic compound. Indeed, motility patterns in scleroderma patients were chaotic and non-propagative, but – after octreotide was given – became well coordinated, aborally directed and nearly as intense as in healthy volunteers [127]. A 3-week treatment with the drug was able to achieve a significant reduction in symptoms such as abdominal pain, bloating, nausea and vomiting. Additionally, there was an improvement in bacterial overgrowth, as objectively measured by breath hydrogen test [127].

A thorough analysis of the effects of octreotide on GI pressure profiles [128] confirmed that it induces a small activity front followed by motor quiescence in both healthy subjects and patients with functional or organic GI disorders and showed an inhibition of antral motility, thus suggesting the drug not to be effective in gastroparesis. A subsequent study [129] demonstrated that octreotide accelerates initial gastric emptying, inhibits small bowel transit, leaving unaltered the colonic transit. While these data support the use of the drug in diarrheal states, they do not provide a rationale for using octreotide to treat small bowel stasis syndromes. The use of this synthetic peptide in GI motor disturbances needs therefore to be further evaluated before any recommendation for clinical practice be given.

Leuprolide

Leuprolide acetate (Lupron®) is a gonadotropin-releasing hormone (GnRH) agonist, which will inhibit ovulatory cycle-changes in circulating concentrations of the gonadal hormones in women with gastroparesis and as a result may improve their symptom complex when compared with placebo treatment. The enthusiasm for this approach to therapy is based on the observation that 90 % of patients with gastroparesis are women and that 90 % of these women are under the age of 45 and hence are premenopausal. In some patients, symptoms start with intermittent cycles of nausea and/or vomiting, bloating or distension. Some patients may be able to correlate the stages of the menstrual cycle. Typically, it is in the luteal phase of the cycle where symptoms are worse, that is, the second half of the cycle, particularly before the onset of menses. With this theory in mind, the hypothesis would be that the symptom complex in women occurring at this stage in the post-ovulatory phase of the menstrual cycle would be influenced by higher concentrations of serum progesterone and relaxin. Therefore, it may be reasonable to investigate if inhibition of this post-ovulatory hormone environment could decrease symptoms of gastroparesis, particularly the cyclical components of nausea and vomiting which over time tend to become more continuous.

There was one early publication by Mathias *et al.* [130] suggesting that, when given for 6 months (0.5 mg subcutaneously) in patients with severe GI motor dysfunction, there was a dramatic improvement in abdominal pain, nausea and vomiting. This has raised the spectrum that this approach of having a GnRH agonist could influence all areas of intestinal smooth muscle abnormalities and would benefit not only the upper GI tract but also be appropriate for IBS [131]. The same group [132] performed a double-blind, placebo controlled study in patients with moderate to severe functional bowel disease. After administration of a long-acting formulation (Lupron® Depot, 3.75 mg monthly) for 3 months, there was a progressive and significant improvement in scores for nausea, vomiting, bloating and early satiety. In the long-term maintenance on subcutaneous leuprolide symptoms improved more than in the short-term treatment [133].

A recent investigation, using myoelectric techniques in rats [134], showed that both leuprolide and ovariectomy modify the intestinal motility pattern, thus suggesting that reproductive hormones have a significant effect on GI motility. Whatever the mechanism of action (affecting GI motility or visceral perception), large and appropriate controlled clinical trials are needed to establish the efficacy and safety of leuprolide in the management of GI motility disorders.

Conclusions

It is now well established that numerous clinical syndromes may be related to motor abnormalities of the upper and/or lower GI motility. Drugs enhancing GI motility and coordination are now available and several new ones are being developed. Further work is needed to determine the predictive value of objective abnormalities for the efficacy of a drug in the individual patient. This is the crucial point to define a rational strategy in clinical practice, especially to establish if functional investigation is needed before a prokinetic drug be given.

Acknowledgements

I am indebted with Dr. Paolo Frati for his invaluable help during the preparation of the manuscript.

References

1. Reynolds JC. Prokinetic agents: a key in the future of gastroenterology. *Gastroenterol Clin North Am* 1989; 18: 437-57.
2. Bertaccini G, Coruzzi G. Recent drugs in gastroenterology. In: Dobrilla G, Liguory C, Misiewicz G, eds. *Current therapy of gastrointestinal disorders*. Verona, New York: Cortina International/Raven Press, 1982: 19-27.
3. Bertaccini G, Coruzzi G. Compounds capable of affecting gastro-esophageal motility. In: Cheli R, Bovero E, Pandolfo N, eds. *Gastric motility. A physiological and pharmacological approach*. Verona, New York: Cortina International/Raven Press, 1988: 110-3.
4. Burks TF. Actions of pharmacological agents on gastrointestinal function. In: Kumar D, Wingate D, eds. *An illustrated guide to gastrointestinal motility*, 2nd ed. Edinburgh: Churchill Livingstone, 1993: 144-61.
5. Hartshorne DJ. Biochemistry of the contractile process in smooth muscle. In: Johnson LR, ed. *Physiology of the gastrointestinal tract*, 2nd ed. New York: Raven Press, 1987: 432-82.
6. Bourne HR, Roberts JM. Drug receptors and pharmacodynamics. In: Katzung BG, ed. *Basic and clinical pharmacology*, 4th ed. Norwalk: Appleton and Lange, 1989: 10-28.
7. Scarpignato C. Pharmacological bases of the medical treatment of gastroesophageal reflux disease. *Dig Dis Sci* 1988; 6: 117-48.
8. Harrington RA, Hamilton CW, Brogden RN, Linkewich JA, Romankiewicz JA, Heel RC. Metoclopramide. An updated review of its pharmacological properties and clinical use. *Drugs* 1983; 25: 451-94.
9. Scarpignato C, Guslandi M. Metoclopramide: is there still a place in the treatment of gastroesophageal reflux disease? *Front Gastrointest Res* 1992; 20: 17-29.
10. Brogden RN, Carmine AA, Heel RC, Speight TM, Avery GS. Domperidone. A review of its pharmacological activity, pharmacokinetics and therapeutic efficacy in the symptomatic treatment of chronic dyspepsia and as an antiemetic. *Drugs* 1982; 24: 360-400.
11. Guslandi M. Antiemetic properties of L-sulpiride. *Minerva Med* 1990; 81: 855-60.
12. McCallum RW, Prakash C, Campoli-Richards DM, Goa KL. Cisapride. A preliminary review of its pharmacodynamic and pharmacokinetic properties, and therapeutic use as a prokinetic agent in gastrointestinal motility disorders. *Drugs* 1988; 36: 652-81.
13. Wiseman Lynda R, Faulds D. Cisapride. An updated review of its pharmacology and therapeutic efficacy as a prokinetic agent in gastrointestinal motility disorders. *Drugs* 1994; 47: 116-52.
14. Van Nueten JM, Schuurkes JAJ. Development of a gastrointestinal prokinetic: pharmacology of cisapride. *Front Gastrointest Res* 1992; 20: 54-63.
15. Talley NJ, Phillips SF, Haddad A, Miller LJ, Twomey C, Zinsmeister AR, MacCarty RL, Ciociola A. GR 38082F (Ondansetron), a selective 5HT3 receptor antagonist, slows colonic transit in healthy man. *Dig Dis Sci* 1990; 35: 477-80.
16. Boeckxstaens GE, Pelckmans PA, Rampart M, Bogers JJ, Verbeuren TJ, Herman AG, Van-Maercke YM. Pharmacological characterization of 5-hydroxytryptamine receptors in the canine terminal ileum and ileocolonic junction. *J Pharmacol Exp Ther* 1990; 254: 652-8.
17. Schuurkes JAJ. Facilitation of acetylcholine release via serotonin receptors: effect of cisapride? In: Heading RC, Wood JD, ed. *Gastrointestinal dysmotility: focus on cisapride*. New York: Raven Press, 1992: 107-15.
18. Tonini M. An appraisal of the action of cisapride and other substituted benzamide prokinetics on myenteric neurons. In: Heading RC, Wood JD, ed. *Gastrointestinal dysmotility: focus on cisapride*, New York: Raven Press, 1992: 85-91.
19. Tari A, Sumii K, Yoshihara M, Ohgoshi H, Teshima H, Fukuhara I, Haruma K, Kajiyama G, Tanaka K, Mijoshi A. Effect of cisapride on the concentrations of beta-endorphin-like immunoreactivity and substance P-like immunoreactivity in the rat gastrointestinal tract. *Biochem Biophys Res Commun* 1987; 147: 1162-9.

20. Peteers TL. Effects of cisapride on gastrointestinal hormones. In: Heading RC, Wood JD, eds. *Gastrointestinal dysmotility: focus on cisapride*. New York: Raven Press, 1992: 117-25.
21. Schuurkes JAJ, Van Nueten JM. Domperidone improves myogenically transmitted antroduodenal coordination by blocking dopaminergic receptor sites. *Scand J Gastroenterol* 1984; 10 (Suppl 94): 101-10.
22. Reynolds JC, Putnam PE. Prokinetic Agents. *Gastroenterol Clin North Am* 1992; 21: 567-96.
23. Corinaldesi R, Stanghellini V, Tosetti C, Rea E, Corbelli C, Marengo M, Monetti N, Barbara L. The effect of different dosage schedules of cisapride on gastric emptying in idiopathic gastroparesis. *Eur J Clin Pharmacol* 1993; 44: 429-32.
24. Bertaccini G. Peptides: gastrointestinal hormones. In: Bertaccini G, ed. *Handbook of experimental pharmacology*, vol. 59/II. Heidelberg: Springer Verlag, 1982: 11-83.
25. Docray GJ. Physiology of enteric neuropeptides. In: Johnson LR, ed. *Physiology of the gastrointestinal tract*, 2nd ed. New York: Raven Press, 1987: 41-66.
26. Bruley des Varannes S, Cloarec D, Dubois A, Galmiche JP. Cholécystokinine et ses antagonistes: effets sur la motricité digestive. *Gastroenterol Clin Biol* 1991; 15: 744-57.
27. Resin H, Stern DH, Sturdevant RAL, Isenberg JI. Effect of the C-terminal octapeptide of cholecystokinin on lower esophageal sphincter pressure in man. *Gastroenterology* 1973; 64: 946-9.
28. Ledeboer ML, Masclee AAM, Batstra M, Lamers CBHW. Effect of cholecystokinin on transient lower esophageal sphincter relaxations. *Gastroenterology* 1993; 104: A539.
29. Scarpignato C, Varga G, Corradi C. Effect of CCK and its antagonists on gastric emptying. *J Physiol* (Paris) 1993; 87: 291-300.
30. Scarpignato C: Cholecystokinin antagonists and motilides: pharmacology and potential in the treatment of gastroesophageal reflux disease and other digestive motor disorders. *Front Gastrointest Res* 1992; 20: 90-128.
31. D'Amato M, Makovec F, Rovati LC. Potential clinical applications of CCK_A-receptor antagonists in gastroenterology. *Drug News Perspectiv* 1994; 7: 87-95.
32. Lotti VJ, Chang RSL. A new potent and selective non-peptide gastrin antagonist and brain cholecystokinin receptor (CCK-B) ligand: L-365,260. *Eur J Pharmacol* 1989; 162: 273-80.
33. Katschinski M, Koppelberg T, Wank U, Adler G, Rovati L, Arnold R. CCK plays a role as a physiological regulator of human esophageal motility. *Gastroenterology* 1990; 98: A365.
34. Buéno L, Fioramonti J. Drug effects on gastric emptying in animal models depend on the nature of test meals used. *Am J Physiol* 1988; 254: G637.
35. Gue M, Fioramonti J, Buéno L. Influence of stress on gastric emptying depends on the nature of meals, stressors, and animal species. *J Gastrointest Motil* 1990; 2: 18-22.
36. Liberge M, Riviere PMJ, Buéno L. Influence of enkephalinase inhibitors on gastric emptying in mice depends on the nature of the meal. *Life Sci* 1988; 42: 2047-53.
37. Meyer BM, Werth BA, Beglinger C, Hildebrand P, Jansen JBMJ, Zach D, Rovati LC, Stalder GA. Role of cholecystokinin in regulation of gastrointestinal motor functions. *Lancet* 1989; ii: 12-5.
38. Fried M, Erlacher URS, Schwizer W, Löchner C, Koerfer J, Beglinger C, Jansen JB, Lamers CB, Harder F, Bischof-Delaloye A, Stalder GA, Rovati L. Role of cholecystokinin in the regulation of gastric emptying and pancreatic enzyme secretion in humans. *Gastroenterology* 1991; 101: 503-11.
39. Corazziari E, Ricci R, Biliotti D, Bontempo I, De'Medici A, Pallotta N, Torsoli A. Oral administration of loxiglumide (CCK antagonist) inhibits postprandial gallbladder contraction without affecting gastric emptying. *Dig Dis Sci* 1990; 35: 50-4.
40. Liddle RA, Gertz BJ, Kanayama S, Beccaria L, Coker LD, Turnbull TA, Morita ET. Effects of a novel cholecystokinin (CCK) receptor antagonist, MK-329, on gallbladder contraction and gastric emptying. Implications for the physiology of CCK. *J Clin Invest* 1989; 84: 1220-5.
41. Cantor P, Mortensen PE, Myhre J, Gjorup I, Worning H, Stahl E, Survill TT. The effect of the cholecystokinin receptor antagonist MK-329 on meal-stimulated pancreaticobiliary output in humans. *Gastroenterology* 1992; 102: 1742-51.

42. Egberts E, Johnson A. The effect of cholecystokinin on human taenia coli. *Digestion* 1977; 15: 217-22.
43. Snape W Jr, Carlson G, Cohen S. Human colonic myoelectric activity in response to prostigmin and the gastrointestinal hormones. *Am J Dig Dis* 1977; 22: 881-7.
44. Snape W Jr. Interaction of the octapeptide of cholecystokinin and gastrin I with bethanechol in the stimulation of feline colonic smooth muscle. *Gastroenterology* 1983; 84: 58-62.
45. Renny A, Snape WJ, Sun E, London R, Cohen S. Role of cholecystokinin in the gastrocolic response to a fat meal. *Gastroenterology* 1983; 85: 17-21.
46. Meier R, Thumshirn M, Meyer B, Rovati LC, Gyr K, Beglinger C. Treatment of chronic constipation in geriatric patients with loxiglumide (LOX), a cholecystokinin antagonist. *Gastroenterology* 1990; 98: A374.
47. Jehle EC, Blum AL, Fried M. Role of cholecystokinin in the regulation of basal colonic motility and the gastrocolic response. *Gastroenterology* 1990; 98: A361.
48. McIntosh CHS, Brown JC. Motilin: isolation, secretion, actions and pathophysiology. *Front Gastrointest Res* 1990; 17: 307-52.
49. Bormans V, Peeters TL, Vantrappen G. Motilin receptors in rabbit stomach and small intestine. *Regul Peptides* 1986; 15: 143-53.
50. Peeters TL, Bormans V, Matthijs G, Vantrappen G. Comparison of the biological activity of canine and porcine motilin in rabbit. *Regul Peptides* 1986; 15: 333-9.
51. Louie DS, Owyang C. Motilin receptors on isolated gastric smooth muscle cells. *Am J Physiol* 1988; 254: G210-G216.
52. Tomomasa T, Kuruome T, Arai H. Erythromycin induces migrating motor complex in human gastrointestinal tract. *Dig Dis Sci* 1986; 31: 157-61.
53. Kondo Y, Torii K, Itoh Z. Erythromycin and its derivatives with motilin-like biological activities inhibit the specific binding of ^{125}I-motilin to duodenal muscle. *Biochem Biophys Res Commun* 1988; 150: 877-82.
54. Peeters T, Matthijs G, Depoortere I. Erythromycin is a motilin receptor agonist. *Am J Physiol* 1989; 257: G470-G474.
55. Michopoulos S, Chaussade S, Guerre J. Effet de l'erythromycine (ERY) sur la motricité oesophagienne chez l'homme normal. *Gastroenterol Clin Biol* 1990; 14 (2bis): 44A.
56. Janssens J, Vantrappen G, Annese V, Peeters TL, Tijskens G, Rekoumis G. Effect of erythromycin on LES function and esophageal body contractility. *Gastroenterology* 1990: 98: A64.
57. Chaussade S, Michopoulos S, Kahan A, Samama J, Danel B, Amor B, Menkès CJ, Guerre J, Couturier D. Effets de l'érythromycine (ERY), un agoniste de la motiline, sur la motricité œsophagienne chez des patients presentant une sclérodermie systémique (S.S.). *Gastroenterol Clin Biol* 1991; 15 (2bis): A35.
58. Dalton CB, DeVore MS, Smout AJPM, Castell DO. The effect of erythromycin (Ery) on lower esophageal sphincter pressure (LESP) and esophageal motility. *Gastroenterology* 1990; 98: A342.
59. Champion G, Singh S, Nellans H, Richter JE. Erythromycin – from acne to acid reflux? *Gastroenterology* 1991; 100: A41.
60. Harrison ME, Ruzkowski CJ, Young MF, Sanowski RA. Erythromycin improves gastric emptying and esophageal motility without affecting gastroesophageal reflux. *Gastroenterology* 1991; 100: A80.
61. Pfeiffer A, Wendl B, Pehl C, Kaess H. Effect of erythromycin on gastroesophageal reflux. *Gastroenterol Clin Biol* 1991; 15: 561-2.
62. Zara GP, Thompson HH, Pilot MA, Ritchie HD. Effects of erythromycin on gastrointestinal tract motility. *J Antimicrob Chemother* 1985; 16 (Suppl A): 175-9.
63. Zara GP, Qin XY, Pilot MA, Thompson H, Maskell J. Response of the human gastrointestinal tract to erythromycin. *J Gastrointest Motil* 1991; 3: 26-31.

64. Janssens J, Peeters TL, Vantrappen G, Tack J, Urbain JL, De Roo M, Muls E, Bouillon R. Improvement of gastric emptying in diabetic gastroparesis by erythromycin. *N Engl J Med* 1990; 322: 1028-31.
65. Pouliquen B, Bizais Y, Murat A, Galmiche JP. L'érythromycine accélère de façon spectaculaire la vidange gastrique (VG) des patients atteints de gastroparésie diabétique (GP). *Gastroenterol Clin Biol* 1990; 14 (2bis): 47A.
66. Richards RD, Davenport K, McCallum RW. The treatment of idiopathic and diabetic gastroparesis with acute intravenous and chronic oral erythromycin. *Am J Gastroenterol* 1993; 88: 203-7.
67. Wadhwa NK, Atkins H, Cabralda T. Intraperitoneal erythromycin for gastroparesis. *Ann Intern Med* 1991; 114: 912.
68. Urbain JLC, Vantrappen G, Janssens J, Van Cutsem E, Peeters T, De Roo M. Intravenous erythromycin dramatically accelerates gastric emptying in gastroparesis diabeticorum and normals and abolishes the emptying discrimination between solids and liquids. *J Nucl Med* 1990; 31: 1490-3.
69. Dull JS, Raufman JP, Zakia MD, Strashun A, Straus EW. Successful treatment of gastroparesis with erythromycin in a patients with progressive systemic sclerosis. *Am J Med* 1990; 89: 528-30.
70. Mantides A, Xynos E, Crhysos E, Georgopoulos N, Vassilakis JS. The effect of erythromycin in gastric emptying of solids and hypertonic liquids in healthy subjects. *Am J Gastroenterol* 1993; 88: 198-202.
71. Prather CM, Camilleri M, Thomforde GM, Forstrom LA, Zinsmeister AR. Gastric axial forces in experimentally delayed and accelerated gastric emptying. *Am J Physiol Gastrointest Liver Physiol* 1993; 264: G928-G934.
72. Annese V, Janssens J, Vantrappen G, Tack J, Peeters TL, Willemse P, Van Cutsem E. Erythromycin accelerates gastric emptying by inducing antral contractions and improved gastroduodenal coordination. *Gastroenterology* 1992; 102: 823-8.
73. Richards RD, Davenport KG, Hurm KD, Wimbish WR, McCallum RW. Acute and chronic treatment of gastroparesis with erythromycin. *Gastroenterology* 1990; 80: A385.
74. Camilleri M. Appraisal of medium- and long-term treatment of gastroparesis and chronic intestinal dysmotility. *Am J Gastroenterol* 1994; 89: 1769-74.
75. Ruppin H, Sturm G, Westhoff D, Domschke S, Domschke W, Wunsch E, Demling I. Effect of 13-Nle-motilin on small intestinal transit time in healthy subjects. *Scand J Gastroenterol* 1976; 11 (Suppl 39): 85-8.
76. Ruppin H, Soergel KH, Dodds JW, *et al*. Effects of the interdigestive motor complex (IMC) and 13-norleucine motilin (NLEM) on fasting intestinal flow rate and velocity in man. *Gastroenterology* 1979; 76: 1231.
77. Lehtola J, Jauhonen P, Kesaniemi A, Wikberg-R, Gordin A. Effect of erythromycin on the oro-caecal transit time in man. *Eur J Clin Pharmacol* 1990; 39: 555-8.
78. Depoortere I, Peeters TL, Vantrappen G. Motilin receptors in the colon of the rabbit. *Gastroenterology* 1990: 98: A345.
79. Hasler A, Heldsinger A, Soudah H, Owyang C. Erythromycin promotes colonic transit in humans: mediation via motilin receptors. *Gastroenterology* 1990; 98: A358.
80. Bassotti G, Betti C, Imbimbo BP, Pelli MA, Morelli A. Erythromycin and edrophonium chloride do not stimulate colonic propagated activity in chronically constipated subjects. *Gastroenterology* 1991; 100: A419.
81. Bonacini M, Quiason S, Gaddis M, Reynolds M, Pemberton LB, Smith OJ. Therapy of postoperative ileus with intravenous erythromycin: preliminary results of a double blind placebo-controlled study. *Gastroenterology* 1991; 100: A423.
82. Schippers E, Hölscher AH, Bollschweiler E, Siewert JR. Return of interdigestive motor complex after abdominal surgery. End of postoperative ileus? *Dig Dis Sci* 1991; 36: 621-6.
83. Miller SM, O'Dorisio TM, Thomas FB, Mekhjian HS. Erythromycin exerts a prokinetic effect in patients with chronic idiopathic intestinal pseudo-obstruction. *Gastroenterology* 1990: 98: A375.

84. Omura S, Tsuzuki K, Sunazuka T, Marui S, Toyoda H, Inatomi N, Itoh Z. Macrolides with gastrointestinal motor stimulating activity. *J Med Chem* 1987; 30: 1941-3.
85. Itoh Z, Omura S. Motilide, a new family of macrolide compounds mimicing motilin. *Dig Dis Sci* 1987; 32: 915.
86. Depoortere I, Peeters TL, Matthijs G, et al. Structure-activity relation of erythromycin-related macrolides in inducing contractions and in displacing bound motilin in rabbit duodenum. *J Gastrointest Motility* 1989; 1: 150-59.
87. Peeters T. Erythromycin and other macrolides as prokinetic agents. *Gastroenterology* 1993; 105: 1886-99.
88. Depoortere I, Peeters T, Vantrappen G. The erythromycin derivative EM-523 is a potent motilin agonist in man and in rabbit. *Peptides* 1990; 11: 515-9.
89. Sakai T, Satoh M, Sano Y, Fujikura K, Koyama H, Itoh Z, Ohmura S. EM574, one of the motilides acts as a motilin agonist on human stomach motilin receptors: *in vitro* demonstrations. *Gastroenterology* 1993; 104: A574.
90. Hanyu N, Aoki T, Furukawa Y, Ohira Y, Morita S, Kajimoto T, Aoki H, Fukuda S, Shiga Y, Tanaka J. Effect of (Leu^{13})-motilin, a motilin derivative, on GI motility in normal subjects. *Gastroenterology* 1993; 104: A518).
91. Nellans HN, Petersen AC, Lartey PA, Peeters TL, Faghih R, Borre A, Seifert T, Hoffman D, Marsh K. Erythromycin derivative, A-81229: a gastrointestinal prokinetic agent. *Gastroenterology* 1994; 106: A547.
92. Takanashi H, Yogo K, Ozaki K, Ikuta M, Akima M, Koga H, Nabata H. Motilin agonistic activities and properties of GM-611, a novel acid-stable erythromycin A derivative. *Gastroenterology* 1994; 106: A575.
93. Greenwood B, Dieckman D, Kirst HA, Gidda JS. Effects of LY267108, an erythromycin analogue derivative, on lower esophageal sphincter function in the cat. *Gastroenterology* 1994; 106: 624-8.
94. Eeckhout C, Fioramonti J, Reling P, Hoeltje D, Bueno L. Comparative effects of erythromycin and a new erythromycin derivative, KC 11458, on postprandial gallbladder emptying in dogs. *Neurogastroenterol Motility* 1994; 6: 161A.
95. Macielag MJ, Gregory RL, Depoortere I, Florance J, Peeters TL, Ward J KimDettelback J, Galdes A. The motilin analog, OHM-11638, induces phase III-like contractions of the upper gut and enhances gastric emptying in the conscious dog. *Gastroenterology* 1995; 108: A642.
96. Maes B, Geypens B, Luypaerts A, Ghoos Y, Rutgeerts P. ABT-229, a new motilin agonist increases gastric emptying of solids in man. *Gastroenterology* 1996; 110: A710.
97. Costall B, Naylor RJ. 5-hydroxytryptamine: new receptors and novel drugs for gastrointestinal motor disorders. *Scand J Gastroenterol* 1990; 25: 769-87.
98. Fernandez AG, Massingham R. Peripheral receptor populations involved in the regulation of gastrointestinal motility and the pharmacological actions of metoclopramide-like drugs. *Life Sci* 1985; 36: 1-14.
99. Fozard JR. 5-HT$_3$ receptors and cytotoxic drug-induced vomiting. *Trends Pharmacol Sci* 1987; 8: 44-5.
100. Gamse R, Buchheit KH. 5-HT$_3$ receptor antagonists: pharmacology and potential in the treatment of gastroesophageal reflux disease. *Front Gastrointest Res* 1992; 20: 81-9.
101. Akkermans LMA, Vos A, Hoekstra A, Roelofs JMM, Horowitz M. Effect of ICS 205-930 (a specific 5-HT$_3$ receptor antagonist) on gastric emptying of a solid meal in normal subjects. *Gut* 1988; 29: 1249-52.
102. McCallum RW, Mittal RK, Sluss J. Effect of ICS 205-930, a potential prokinetic agent, on upper gastrointestinal motility in normal subjects. *Gastroenterology* 1989; 96: A332.
103. Stacher G, Bergmann H, Granser-Vacariu GV, Wiesnagrotzki S, Wenzel-Abatzi Th-A, Gaupmann G, Kugi A, Steinringer H, Schneider C, Höbart J. Lack of systematic effects of the 5-hydroxytryptamine$_3$ receptor antagonist ICS 205-930 on gastric emptying and antral motor activity in patients with primary anorexia nervosa. *Br J Clin Pharmacol* 1991; 32: 685-90.

104. Talley NJ, Phillips SF, Haddad A, Miller LJ, Twomey C, Zinsmeister AR, Ciocola A. Effect of selective 5-HT$_3$ antagonist (GR 38032F) on small intestinal transit and release of gastrointestinal peptides. *Dig Dis Sci* 1989; 34: 1511-5.
105. Gore S, Gilmore IT, Haigh CG, Morris AI. Specific 5-hydroxytryptamine receptor (type 3) antagonists GR38032F slows colonic transit. *Gastroenterology* 1989; 96: A178.
106. Nielsen OH, Hvid-Jacobsen K, Lund P, Lanholz E. Gastric emptying and subjective symptoms of nausea: lack of effects of a 5-hydroxytryptamine-3 antagonist ondansetron on gastric emptying in patients with gastric stasis syndrome. *Digestion* 1990; 46: 89-96.
107. Stacher G, Steiner G, Gaupmann G, Stacher-Janotta G, Schneider C, Steinringer H. Effects of the 5-HT$_3$ antagonist, ICS 205-930, on oesophageal motor activity and on lower oesophageal sphincter pressure: a double-blind crossover study. *Hepatogastroenterology* 1990; 37 (Suppl 2): 118-21.
108. McCallum RW, Mittal RK, Sluss J. Effect of ICS 205-930, a potential gastrokinetic agent, on upper gastrointestinal (GI) motility in normal subjects. *Gastroenterology* 1989; 96: A332.
109. von der Ohe MR, Hanson RB, Camilleri M. Serotoninergic mediation of postprandial colonic tone and phasic responses in humans. *Gut* 1994; 35: 536-41.
110. Scolapio JS, Camilleri M, von der Ohe MR, Hanson RB. Ascending colon response to feeding: evidence for a 5-hydroxytryptamine-3 mechanism. *Scand J Gastroenterol* 1995; 30: 562-7.
111. von der Ohe MR, Camilleri M, Kvols LK. A 5-HT$_3$ antagonist corrects the postprandial colonic hypertonic response in carcinoid diarrhea. *Gastroenterology* 1994; 106: 1184-9.
112. Sanger GJ. Increased gut cholinergic activity and antagonism of 5-hydroxytryptamine M-receptors by BRL-24924: potential clinical importance of BRL-24924. *Br J Pharmacol* 1987; 91: 77-87.
113. Yoshida N, Omoya H, Oka M, Furukawa K, Ito T, Karasawa T. AS-4370, a novel gastrokinetic agent free of dopamine D-2 receptor antagonist properties. *Arch Int Pharmacodyn Ther* 1989; 300: 51-67.
114. Fernandez AG, Puig J, Gristwood RW, Berga P. Pancopride: a novel 5-HT$_3$ antagonist with potent antiemetic action. *Eur J Pharmacol* 1990; 183: 1214.
115. Turconi M, Schiantarelli P, Borsini F, Rizzi CA, Ladinsky H, Donetti A. Azabicycloalkyl: interaction with serotonergic 5-HT$_3$ and 5-HT$_4$ receptors and potential therapeutic implications. *Drugs Future* 1991; 16: 1011-26.
116. Gullikson GW, Virina MA, Loeffler RF, Yang DC, Goldstin B, Flynn DL, Moormann AE. Gastrointestinal motility responses to the S and R enantiomers of zacopride, a 5-HT$_4$ and 5-HT$_3$ antagonist. *Drug Dev Res* 1992; 26: 405-17.
117. Flynn DL, Zabrowski DL, Becker DP, Nosal R, Villamil CI, Gullikson GW, Moummi C, Yang DC. SC-53116: The first selective agonist at the newly identified serotonin 5-HT$_4$ receptor subtype. *J Med Chem* 1992; 35: 1486-9.
118. Clark RD, Miller AB, Berger J, Repke DB, Weinhardt KK, Kowalczyk BA, Eglen RM, Bonhaus DW, Lee CH, Michel AD, Smith WL, Wong EHF. 2-(Quinuclidin-3-yl)pyrido[4,3-b]indol-1-ones and isoquinolin-1-ones. Potent conformationally restricted 5-HT$_3$ receptor antagonists. *J Med Chem* 1993; 36: 2645-57.
119. Buchheit KH, Gamse R, Giger R, Hoyer D, Klein F, Kloppner E, Pfannkuche HJ, Mattes H. The serotonin 5-HT$_4$ receptor. 2. Structure – activity studies of the indole carbazimidamide class of agonist. *J Med Chem* 1995; 38: 2331-8.
120. Gullikson GW, Loeffler RF, Virina MA. Relationship of serotonin-3 receptor antagonist activity to gastric emptying and motor-stimulating actions of prokinetic drugs in dogs. *J Pharmacol Exp Ther* 1991; 258: 103-10.
121. Tonini M, Rizzi CA, Manzo L, Onori L. Novel enteric 5-HT$_4$ receptors and gastrointestinal prokinetic action. *Pharmacol Res* 1991; 24: 5-14.
122. Ormsbee HS, Koehler SI, Telford GL. Somatostatin inhibits motilin-induced interdigestive contractile activity in the dog. *Dig Dis Sci* 1978; 23: 781-8.

123. Hostein J, Janssens J, Vantrappen G, Peteers T, Vandeweerd M, Leman G. Somatostatin induces ectopic activity fronts of the migrating motor complex via a local intestinal mechanism. *Gastroenterology* 1984; 87: 1004-8.
124. Peeters T, Janssens J, Vantrappen G. Somatostatin and the interdigestive migrating motor complex in man. *Regul Peptides* 1983; 5: 209-17.
125. Scarpignato C. Octreotide, the synthetic long-acting somatostatin analogue: pharmacological profile. *Prog Basic Clin Pharmacol* 1995; 10: 54-72.
126. Peeters T, Romanski KW, Janssens J, Vantrappen G. Effect of the long-acting somatostatin analogue SMS 201-995 on small intestinal interdigestive motility in the dog. *Scand J Gastroenterol* 1988; 23: 769-74.
127. Soudah HC, Hasler WL, Owyang C. Effect of octreotide on intestinal motility and bacterial overgrowth in scleroderma. *N Engl J Med* 1991; 325: 1461-7.
128. Haruma K, Wiste JA, Camilleri M. Effect of octreotide on gastrointestinal pressure profiles in health and in functional and organic gastrointestinal disorders. *Gut* 1994; 35: 1064-9.
129. van der Ohe MR, Camilleri M, Thomforde GM, Klee GG. Differential regional effects of octreotide on human gastrointestinal motor function. *Gut* 1995; 36: 743-8.
130. Mathias JR, Ferguson KL, Clench MH. Debilitating « functional » bowel disease controlled by leuprolide acetate, gonadotropin-releasing hormone (GnRH) analog. *Dig Dis Sci* 1989; 34: 761-6.
131. Wood JD. Efficacy of leuprolide in treatment of the irritable bowel syndrome. *Dig Dis Sci* 1994; 39: 1153-4.
132. Mathias JR, Clench MH, Reeves-Darby VG, Fox LM, Hsu PH, Roberts PH, Smith LL, Stiglich NJ. Effect of leuprolide acetate in patients with moderate to severe functional bowel disease. Double-blind, placebo-controlled study. *Dig Dis Sci* 1994; 39: 1155-62.
133. Mathias JR, Clench MH, Roberts PH, Reeves-Darby VG. Effect of leuprolide acetate in patients with functional bowel disease. Long-term follow-up after double-blind, placebo controlled study. *Dig Dis Sci* 1994; 39: 1163-70.
134. Khanna R, Browne RM, Heiner AD, Clench MH, Mathias JR. Leuprolide acetate affects intestinal motility in female rats before and after ovariectomy. *Am J Physiol* 1992; 262: G185-G190.

Advances in medical therapy of inflammatory bowel disease

P. Rutgeerts, S. Vermeire

Department of Medicine, University Hospital, 3000 Leuven, Belgium

Summary

The main advances in the treatment of inflammatory bowel disease concern management of intractable and steroid dependent Crohn's disease and ulcerative colitis. Immunosuppression is now used worldwide with good efficacy and acceptable short-term safety. IV cyclosporin is an alternative to colectomy in the presence of acute ulcerative colitis not responsive to glucocorticosteroids but is not yet an alternative on the long-term. Azathioprine, 6-mercaptopurine and methotrexate are important drugs for the long-term management of Crohn's disease whereas their role in ulcerative colitis is less well defined. The future seems to lie in therapy with immunomodulating agents including antibodies against TNFα and interleukin 10. For the acute treatment of ileocolonic Crohn's disease, budesonide turns out to be a safe alternative to standard glucocorticosteroids. The role of antibiotics in the treatment of attacks of Crohn's disease is important but not well defined. Much research is needed to come to an optimal therapy of these puzzling diseases.

Crohn's disease is a more heterogenic disease than ulcerative colitis and is associated with many more systemic problems and complications. For both diseases the severity and extent greatly influence therapeutic decisions which are frequently taken by a team composed of physicians and surgeons. Although ulcerative colitis and Crohn's disease are definitely two different diseases, the pharmacological therapy of both conditions has been remarkably similar in contrast with surgical management. Current therapy with sulphasalazine and 5-ASA formulations has been refined. The greatest advances, however, have occurred in immunosuppression and immunomodulation therapy. Introduction of topically acting glucocorticosteroids and the increasing use of antibiotics are two other important evolutions in the treatment of inflammatory bowel diseases (IBD). We will focus this discussion on those aspects of treatment.

Immunosuppression and immunomodulation therapy in inflammatory bowel disease

Immunosuppression therapy with azathioprine and 6-mercaptapurine is now widely accepted for the treatment of resistant Crohn's disease [1]. Methotrexate may substitute for these drugs in particular therapeutic situations. In ulcerative colitis, cyclosporin therapy has emerged as an important alternative to colectomy.

Cyclosporin therapy in inflammatory bowel disease

Cyclosporin A (CsA) is a potent inhibitor of cell-mediated immunity by blocking the production of IL-2 by T-helper lymphocytes. CsA also inhibits β-cell activation by INFγ. Other leucocytes are not affected. At what level of the mucosal immune system or even of the systemic immune system CsA exerts its action in IBD is not known. When using CsA one should be aware of its toxicity especially renal toxicity, hypertension and infections due to immunosuppression.

Cyclosporin A (CsA) in severe ulcerative colitis

Uncontrolled studies of intravenous CsA in severe ulcerative colitis resistant to high dose IV steroids in a dose of 1-7 mg/kg/day or oral treatment with 5-15 mg/kg/day resulted in a mean response rate of 68 % (125/185 patients) with a maintained response in 42 % of the patients [2]. The efficacy of this treatment was then unequivocally demonstrated by one small but important controlled trial [3] in 20 patients with severe left-sided or extensive ulcerative colitis resistant to high dose IV glucocorticosteroids. Eleven patients received IV CsA 4 mg/kg/day and nine received placebo. After 14 days nine of the eleven patients treated with CsA had improved *versus* none of the nine patients receiving placebo. Five patients who failed on placebo responded on switch to IV cyclosporin. Long-term efficacy of oral maintenance therapy with 8 mg/kg/day for 6 months in these patients was successful in only 45 % of the patients [4]. A non-colectomy « survival » was achieved in 35.5 % after 2.8 years [5].

In another preliminary report, the long-term response was 43 % [6].

The efficacy of IV cyclosporin for the management of severe steroid refractory ulcerative colitis seems established but the problems of safety and especially long-term therapy of these patients are unresolved.

These patients are at risk for cumulative toxicity of IV cyclosporin and high doses of glucocorticosteroids.

Our recent observation [7] that IV cyclosporin without glucocorticosteroids may be effective should stimulate the evaluation of monotherapy with cyclosporin in severe ulcerative colitis.

Data on topical use of cyclosporin enemas in refractory left sided colitis are not really encouraging [2]. The only controlled trial [8] comparing 350 mg/day enema with placebo in left sided ulcerative colitis showed comparable efficacy. Whole blood concentrations of CsA were not detectable.

Cyclosporin in Crohn's disease

The results of cyclosporin in Crohn's disease are definitely less promising than in ulcerative colitis although high dose intravenous therapy has not been tested. Of four large multicenter controlled trials [9-12], only one [9] showed a therapeutic advance of cyclosporin (5-7.5 mg/kg/day) over placebo in active Crohn's disease (response rate 59 % in CsA group and 32 % in the placebo group at three months).

There are uncontrolled data that ulcerative colitis-like Crohn's colitis might respond as well to high dose IV CsA as ulcerative colitis and CsA therefore is proposed by some as « rescue therapy » in short-term management of severe Crohn's disease [13]. It is also claimed to be very efficacious in fistulous disease [14] although some authors did not confirm this [15] and controlled studies are warranted.

Azathioprine and 6-mercaptopurine in inflammatory bowel disease

The value of 6-MP in the treatment of Crohn's disease was established by the pivotal study of Present *et al.* [16]. They showed that the response occurs with a delay of 3-6 months and therefore lacks short-term benefit.

The auhors showed the efficacy for steroid-tapering, improvement of chronically active disease and healing of fistulae. Recent studies have provided interesting new data. Although these drugs are indicated for the treatment of chronic refractory disease, addition of azathioprine to glucocorticosteroids improves the short-term outcome of this drug [17]. The beneficial effect of azathioprine or 6-MP persists at least for a period of four years [18]. Long-term safety of this therapy is acceptable provided that leucocyte counts are measured at regular intervals [19]. It has been claimed that in the presence of neutropenia optimal efficacy of this therapy is achieved but more data are necessary [20]. Our studies have shown that long-term azathioprine may contribute to healing of severe recurrent Crohn's ileitis [21]. The effect of azathioprine and 6-mercaptopurine has not been studied in ulcerative colitis as well as in Crohn's disease. Uncontrolled experience in ulcerative colitis seems less impressive than in Crohn's disease. One controlled trial has documented the maintenance benefit for azathioprine in patients who responded to this therapy for steroid-sparing in ulcerative colitis [22].

Safety remains an important issue with this therapy. Recent reports claim that immunosuppression with these drugs is safe even during pregnancy [23].

Methotrexate in inflammatory bowel disease

The efficacy of immunosuppression with the folic acid inhibitor, methotrexate in the treatment of active refractory Crohn's disease was demonstrated by Kazarek *et al.* [24]. A collaborative North American controlled study [25] showed that parenteral methotrexate 25 mg IV per week allowed steroid withdrawal in 39 % of steroid-dependent patients.

There were more withdrawals for adverse effects in the methotrexate group than in the placebo group. The long-term effect of this therapy and the safety have to be studied.

New immunomodulators in the treatment of inflammatory bowel disease

Progress in understanding of the pathogenesis of Crohn's disease and ulcerative colitis led to these new forms of therapy. At present cytokines including TNFα and IL-1β are considered proinflammatory and interleukin-10 seems to be the main antiinflammatory cytokine. Single infusion of an anti-tumor necrosis factor (anti-TNF) mouse/human chimeric monoclonal antibody (10 or 20 mg/kg) dramatically improved prednisolone-unresponsive Crohn's disease in an open trial in 10 patients at eight weeks with extensive endoscopic healing at 4 weeks [26]. A multicenter controlled trial [27] confirmed the efficacy and safety of this treatment. The dramatic effect on endoscopy and histology was also confirmed [28]. The effect of cA2 in ulcerative colitis seems to be less pronounced [29]. Therapy with cA2 seems safe.

Interleukin-10 infusion also is safe and effective *versus* placebo in patients with steroid refractory Crohn's disease [30]. The optimal dose still has to be determined.

Immunomodulatory therapy in IBD is very promising. A number of trials are ungoing and will define the role of these therapies in the management of Crohn's disease and ulcerative colitis.

Treatment with topically acting glucocorticosteroids in inflammatory bowel disease

The efficacy and safety of topical enema therapy using the new glucocorticosteroid budesonide in distal colitis are already well established. Recent developments in the use of this drug for peroral therapy in Crohn's disease is of great interest. Oral formulations are also under study for the treatment of ulcerative colitis but data are not yet available. We therefore will focus this review on the use of topically acting glucocorticosteroids in Crohn's disease.

In the past years numerous attempts have been made to develop glucocorticosteroids with high topical activity lacking the systemic activity of the drug and hence carrying less side effects.

The ideal topically acting glucocorticosteroid should have sufficient water solubility for a homogeneous distribution in the bowel lumen. A high uptake rate should be combined with sustained binding at the level of the target tissue with deep penetration into the bowel wall. There should be a high affinity for the steroid receptor and high intrinsic activity at this level. Hepatic first pass inactivation should be maximal. Candidate drugs are budesonide, fluticasone propionate and beclomethasone dipropionate.

Budesonide, however, has the best profile since its water solubility is 100 times higher than that of the two latter drugs. Crohn's disease is mostly located in the ileocolonic region of the bowel whereas isolated colonic disease occurs in about 30 % of the patients and isolated proximal small bowel disease is very rare. Therefore formulations used should release the drug at the very site of the diseased bowel.

Entocort® capsules release budesonide in a controlled manner in the ileum resulting in an absorption of 52-79 % in the ileum and the right colon [31]. The drug is largely metabolized on first pass through the liver resulting in a bioavailability of 9-12 %. Preliminary studies indicate that plasma concentrations in patients with active Crohn's disease might be higher than in normal volunteers [32]. The influence of feeding with this preparation on pharmacokinetics seems not important.

Budenofalk® results in absorption of budesonide after 2-4 hours, the rate being influenced by feeding. Measurements of excretion in ileostoma bags showed that 25-37 % of the budesonide of this formulation enters the colon [33].

Clinical trials in active Crohn's disease have been carried out mainly with Entocort® capsules.

Trials with budesonide in ileal and right ileocolonic Crohn's disease

Open trial with Entocort®

Löfberg et al. [34] studied the efficacy and safety of controlled ileal release budesonide in an open uncontrolled trial. Twenty-one patients with active Crohn's disease involving the distal ileum, the ileocecal area or the ascending colon entered the trial. The patients received budesonide CIR in a dose of 3 mg t.d.s. for 12 weeks, followed by tapering to 2 mg t.d.s. for 6 weeks and finally to 1 mg t.d.s. for an additional 6 weeks. Primary variables of efficacy were a modified Crohn's disease activity index (mCDAI), laboratory parameters of activity and plasma cortisol levels. The mean mCDAI level at entry amounted to 268 ($\pm$ 71-sd) and decreased to 146 ($\pm$ 91) at four weeks, 122 ($\pm$ 87) at 12 weeks ($p < 0.001$). There was also a significant decrease of ESR during the study period. Eighteen patients responded favourably during the first 12-week treatment period and 13 completed the trial. No serious side effects occurred. The mean plasma cortisol levels decreased but remained within normal range. Four patients were markedly suppressed on the highest dose of budesonide.

Controlled trials with Entocort®

In a double-blind multicenter Canadian dose finding trial [35], 258 patients were randomly assigned to receive placebo or one of three doses of budesonide - 3,9 or 15 mg daily. The drugs were given in two divided doses in the morning and the evening. The primary outcome measure was clinical remission as defined by a score of 150 or less on the Crohn's activity index. Changes in the quality of life were also assessed with an inflammatory bowel disease questionnaire. Serum corticotropin stimulation tests were also performed. After eight weeks of treatment, remission occurred in 51 % of the patients in the group receiving 9 mg of budesonide (95 % confidence interval, 39 to 63 %), 43 % of those receiving 15 mg (95 % confidence interval, 31 to 55 %) and 33 % of those receiving 3 mg (95 % confidence interval, 21 to 44 %) as compared with 20 % of those receiving placebo (p < 0.001, p = 0.009 and p = 0.13 respectively). Improvements in the quality of life paralleled these remission rates. Location of disease, prior surgical resection, and previous use of corticosteroids did not affect the outcome. Budesonide caused a dose-related reduction in basal and corticotropin-stimulated plasma cortisol concentrations but was not associated with clinically important corticosteroid-related symptoms or other toxic effects.

A European multicenter study group conducted a randomized double-blind 10-week trial [36] comparing the efficacy and safety of an oral controlled-release form of budesonide with the efficacy and safety of prednisolone in 176 patients with active ileal or ileocecal Crohn's disease (88 patients in each treatment group). The dose of budesonide was 9 mg per day for eight weeks and then 6 mg per day for two weeks. The dose of prednisolone was 40 mg per day for two weeks, after which it was gradually reduced to 5 mg per day during the last week. Again the primary outcome parameter was the CDAI score with remission defined as a score of 150 or less. Three objective parameters of inflammation were also assessed including ESR, C-reactive protein and orosomucoid.

At ten weeks, 53 % of the patients treated with budesonide were in remission as compared with 66 % of those treated with prednisolone (p = 0.12). The mean score on the Crohn's disease activity index decreased from 275 to 175 in the budesonide group and from 279 to 136 in the prednisolone group (p = 0.001). ESR, CRP and orosomucoid decreased more in the prednisolone group than in the budesonide group but the difference was significant only for ESR. Corticosteroid-associated side-effects were significantly less common in the budesonide group (29 vs 48 patients, p = 0.003). Two patients in the prednisolone group had serious complications (one had intestinal perforation and one an abdominal wall fistula). The mean morning plasma cortisol concentration was significantly lower in the prednisolone group than in the budesonide group after 4 weeks (p < 0.001) and 8 weeks (p = 0.02) of therapy, but not after 10 weeks.

An International Budesonide study group [37] investigated the efficacy and safety of two different dosage regimens of budesonide, 9 mg once daily (o.m.) in the morning and 4.5 mg twice daily in comparison with prednisolone 40 mg in one dose daily. In this multicenter trial, 177 patients with active Crohn's disease (CDAI > 200) were randomly assigned to one of the three treatments for 12 weeks. The budesonide dose was tapered to 30 mg after two weeks and to 3 mg after 10 weeks.

Prednisolone was tapered to 30 mg after two weeks and then gradually to 5 mg during the last three weeks. Efficacy was measured based on remission rates, with remission being defined as CDAI ≤ 150. During therapy disease activity rapidly decreased in all groups. After two weeks the remission rate amounted to 48 % in the budesonide (o.m.) as compared to 37 % in the prednisolone group. At 8 weeks similar remission rates were observed in the budesonide (o.m.) and prednisolone groups (both 60 %) compared with 42 % in the budesonide b.i.d. group. The proportion of patients with corticosteroid-associated side-effects was not significantly different in the three groups but the proportion of patients with moon face was significantly higher in the prednisolone group. At 8 weeks mean morning plasma cortisol levels were significantly less suppressed in both budesonide groups than in the prednisolone group. Impaired adrenal function as assessed by a short ACTH stimulation test was also significantly more common in the prednisolone group than in the budesonide group.

Budenofalk® versus 6-methylprednisolone

In this study [38], only 67 patients with active Crohn's disease were included. Thirty-four patients were treated with 3 x 3 mg per day of budesonide and 33 with 6-methylprednisolone 48 mg per day with tapering. At eight weeks, 55.9 % of the budesonide patients achieved remission *versus* 72.7 % in the 6-methylprednisolone group. The difference was not significant. There was a greater decrease, although not significant, of the CDAI in the 6-methylprednisolone group than in the budesonide group (BUD: 263 ± 50 to 118 ± 69; M-Pred: 262 ± 81 to 95 ± 61). Steroid related side effects appeared in 28.6 % of the patients in the budesonide group and in 69.7 % in the 6-methylprednisolone group (p = 0.0015).

Budesonide for maintenance therapy of Crohn's disease

During a one-year follow-up study of the European multicentre trial [36], 90 patients with active Crohn's disease in the terminal ileum of the ileocecal area who were in remission (CDAI-score ≤ 150) after 10 weeks treatment with either oral Entocort® or oral prednisolone, were randomised to receive continued treatment with either Entocort® 6 mg or 3 mg daily, or placebo for up to one year in order to prevent relapse [39]. A relapse was defined as an increase of the CDAI-score above 150 points, and at least 60 points above the baseline, or deterioration of the disease that required other treatment.

This double-blind, controlled, randomised trial involved 11 centres in six European countries. The 6 mg group had significantly longer median time to relapse or discontinuation of treatment compared to the placebo group (258 *versus* 92 days; p = 0.02). An adrenocorticotropic hormone (ACTH)-test performed after 3 months was normal in all 13 patients (100 %) remaining in the placebo group at this stage of the study, compared to 19 out of 22 patients (86.4 %) in the Entocort® 3 mg group, and 18 out of 23 patients (78.3 %) in the Entocort® 6 mg group. There were no statistically significant differences between the three treatment groups. Glucocorticosteroid-related side effects were mild (*i.e.* moon-face, acne) and mostly related to previous prednisolone treatment.

A continuation of the Canadian multicentre study [35] of Entocort® *versus* placebo for active Crohn's disease was designed in a similar way to the European maintenance trial. One hundred and five patients with inactive Crohn's disease in the ileum or ileum and proximal colon received continued treatment with either placebo or oral Entocort® 3 or 6 mg daily in a 12-month, double-blind, randomised trial [40].

The Entocort® 6 mg group also fared better in this study, with median time to relapse or discontinuation of therapy of 178 days, *versus* 124 days in the 3 mg group, and 39 days among placebo-treated patients (p = 0.026). However, the rate of relapse did not differ significantly between the three treatment groups after 12 months treatment; 61 % of the patients in the Entocort® 6 mg treatment group had relapsed after 12 months, as compared with 70 % in the Entocort® 3 mg treatment group and 67 % in the placebo group (p = 0.75). The relapse rates at one year were in agreement with the results documented from the European study.

Basal levels of plasma cortisol did not differ between the three study groups during the trial. A dose-dependent reduction in ACTH-stimulated cortisol concentration was found, but was not associated with clinically important steroid-related side effects.

Treatment of attacks of inflammatory bowel disease with antibiotics

Antibiotics are probably the drugs most widely used in the treatment of Crohn's disease.

Still trials are scarce probably also because pharmaceutical companies selling antibiotics are less interested in this patient population. Most data are available for metronidazole which is effective to control mild to moderate Crohn's disease [41, 42] but is the treatment of choice for perianal disease [43]. Metronidazole is also efficacious as prophylaxis for recurrence of Crohn's disease after ileocolonic resection [44]. High dose metronidazole therapy however is associated with many adverse effects.

The combination of ciprofloxacin and metronidazole seems beneficial for the treatment of perianal Crohn's disease [45] as well as for the control of intestinal disease [46].

A recent report [47] on the long-term remission obtained with clarithromycin is of great interest. Whether this effect is due to the activity of this antibiotic against mycobacterium paratuberculosis remains speculative.

References

1. Pearson DC, May GR, Fiek GH, Sutherland LR. Azathioprine and 6-mercaptopurine in Crohn's disease: a metaanalysis. *Ann Intern Med* 1995; 122: 132-42.
2. Sandborn WJ. A critical review of cyclosporine therapy in inflammatory bowel disease. *Inflammatory Bowel Diseases* 1995; 1: 48-63.
3. Lichtiger S, Present DH, Korkbluth A, Gelernt I, Bauer J, Jaller G, Michelassi F, Hanauer S. Cyclosporin in severe ulcerative colitis refractory to steroid therapy. *N Engl J Med* 1994; 330: 1841-5.
4. Kornbluth A, Lichtiger S, Present D, Hanauer S. Long term results of oral cyclosporin in patients with severe ulcerative colitis: a double-blind randomised multicenter trial. *Gastroenterology* 1994; 106: A714.
5. Baert F, Hanauer S. CYA in severe steroid-resistant UC: long-term results of therapy. *Gastroenterology* 1994; 106: A648.
6. Van Gossum A, Schmit A, Adler M, Chiocioli C, Fiasse R, Louwagie P, D'Haens G, Rutgeerts P, Devos M, Reynaert H, Devis G, Belaiche J, Van Outryve M. Administration of cyclosporine in acute severe ulcerative colitis: short-term efficacy and long-term outcome. *Gastroenterology* 1996; 110: A1035.
7. Vermeire S, Rutgeerts P. Cyclosporin monotherapy is effective in the treatment of severe colitis (case report). *Inflammatory Bowel Diseases* 1996; in press.
8. Sandborn WJ, Tremaine WJ, Schroeder KW, Batts KP, Lawson GM, Steiner BL, Harrison JM, Zinmeister AR. A placebo-controlled trial of cyclosporine enemas for mildly to moderately active left-sided ulcerative colitis. *Gastroenterology* 1994; 106: 1429-35.

9. Brynskov J, Freund L, Rasmussen SN. Final report on a placebo-controlled, double-blind, randomized trial of cyclosporin treatment in active chronic Crohn's disease. *Scand J Gastroenterol* 1991; 26: 689-95.
10. Feagan BG, McDonald JWD, Rochon J, Laupacis A, Fedorak RN, Kinnear D, Saibil F, Groll A, Archambault A, Gillies R, Valberg B, Irvina EJ. Low-dose cyclosporine for the treatment of Crohn's disease. *N Engl J Med* 1994; 330: 1846-51.
11. Jewell DP, Lennard-Jones JE, and the cyclosporin study group of Great-Britain and Ireland. Oral cyclosporin for chronic active Crohn's disease: a multicentre controlled trial. *Eur J Gastroenterol Hepatol* 1994; 6: 499-505.
12. Stange EF, Modigliani R, Pena AS, Wood AJ, Feutren G, Smith PR and the European Study Group. European trial of cyclosporine in chronic active Crohn's disease: a 12 month study. *Gastroenterology* 1995; 109: 774-82.
13. Lichtiger S. To use or not to use cyclosporine-A. That is the question. *Inflammatory Bowel Diseases* 1995; 1: 331-4.
14. Hanauer SB, Smith MB. Rapid closure of Crohn's disease fistulas with intravenous cyclosporin A. *Am J Gastroenterol* 1993; 88: 646-9.
15. Markowitz J. Cyclosporine lacks therapeutic efficacy in highly destructive perianal Crohn's disease associated with Crohn's disease (CD). *Am J Gastroenterol* 1993; 88: 1620-4.
16. Present DH, Korelitz BI, Wisch N, Glass JL, Sachar DB, Pasternack BS. Treatment of Cron's disease with 6-mercaptopurine. A long-term randomized double blind study. *N Engl J Med* 1980; 302: 981-7.
17. Ewe K, Press AG, Singe CC, Stufler M, Veberschaer B, Hommel G, Meyer-zum-Buschenfelde KH. Azathioprine combined with prednisolone or monotherapy with prednisolone in active Crohn's disease. *Gastroenterology* 1993; 105: 367-72.
18. Bouhnik Y, Lémann M, Mary JY, Scemama G, Taï R, Matuchansky C, Modigliani R, Rambaud JC. Long term follow-up of patients with Crohn's disease treated with azathioprine or 6-mercaptopurine. *Lancet* 1996; 347: 215-9.
19. Connell WR, Kamm MA, Ritchie JK, Lennard-Jones JE. Bone marrow toxicity caused by azathioprine in inflammatory bowel disease: 27 years of experience. *Gut* 1993; 34: 1081-5.
20. Colonna T, Korelitz BI. The role of leukopenia in the 6-mercaptopurine-induced remission of refractory Crohn's disease. *Am J Gastroenterol* 1994; 89: 362-6.
21. D'Haens G, Peeters M, Geboes K, Rutgeerts P. Azathioprine induces mucosal healing in severe recurrent Crohn's ileitis after surgery. *Gastroenterology* 1995; 108: A809.
22. Hawthorne AB, Logan RFA, Hawkey CJ. Randomized controlled trial of azathioprine withdrawal in ulcerative colitis. *Br Med J* 1992; 305: 20-2.
23. Francella A, Dayan A, Rubin P, Chapman M, Present D. 6-Mercaptopurine (6-MP) is safe therapy for child bearing patients with IBD: a case controlled study. *Gastroenterology* 1996; 110: A909.
24. Kozarek RA, Patterson DJ, Gelfand MD. Methotrexate induces clinical and histological remission in patients with refractory inflammatory bowel disease. *Ann Intern Med* 1989; 110: 353-6.
25. Feagan BG, Rochon J, Fedorak RN, Irvine EJ, Wild G, Sutherland L, Steinhart AH, Greenberg GR, Gillies R, Hopkins M, Hanauer SB, McDonald JWD for the North American Crohn's Study Group Investigators. Methotrexate for the treatment of Crohn's disease. *N Engl J Med* 1995; 332: 292-7.
26. Van Dullemen HN, Van Deventer SJM, Hommes DW, Bijl HA, Jansen J, Tytgat GNJ, Woody J. Treatment of Crohn's disease with anti-tumor necrosis factor chimeric antibody (cA2). *Gastroenterology* 1995; 109: 129-35.
27. Targan SR, Rutgeerts P, Hanauer SB, Van Deventer SJH, Mayer L, Present DH, Braakman TAJ, Woody JN. A multicenter trial of anti-tumor necrosis factor (TNF) antibody (cA2) for the treatment of patients with active Crohn's disease. *Gastroenterology* 1996; 110: A1026.
28. Baert F, D'Haens G, Geboes K, Ectors N, Rutgeerts P. TNF-α antibody therapy causes a fast and dramatic decrease of histologic colonic inflammation in Crohn's disease but not in ulcerative colitis. *Gastroenterology* 1996; 110: A859.

29. Sands BE, Podolsky DK, Tremaine WJ, Sandborne WJ, Rutgeerts PJ, Hanauer SB, Mayer L, Targan SR, De Woody KL, Braakman TAJ, Woody JN. Chimeric monoclonal anti-tumor necrosis factor antibody (cA2) in the treatment of severe steroid refractory ulcerative colitis. *Gastroenterology* 1996; 110: A1008.
30. Van Deventer SJH, Elson CO, Fedorak RN. Safety, tolerance, pharmacokinetics and pharmacodynamics of recombinant interleukin-10 (SCH 52000) in patients with steroid refractory Crohn's disease. *Gastroenterology* 1996; 110: A1034.
31. Edsbäcker S, Wollmer P, Nilsson Å, Nillson M. Pharmacokinetics and gastrointestinal transit of budesonide controlled ileal release (CIR) capsules. *Gastroenterology* 1993; 104: A695.
32. Naber AHJ, Olaison G, Smedh K, Jansen JBMJ, Sjödahl R. Pharmacokinetics of budesonide controlled ileal release capsules in active Crohn's disease. *Gastroenterology* 1996; 110: A977.
33. Moellmann HW, Hochhaus G, Tromm A, Moellmann A, Derendorf H, Barth J, Froehlich P, Ecker KW, Lindemann A. Pharmacokinetics and evaluation of systemic side effects of budesonide after oral administration of modified release capsules in healthy volunteers, ileostoma patients and patients with Crohn's disease. *Gastroenterology* 1996; 110: A972.
34. Löfberg R, Danielsson Å, Salde L. Oral budesonide in active ileal Crohn's disease - a pilot trial with a topically acting steroid. *Aliment Pharmacol Ther* 1993; 7: 611-6.
35. Greenberg GR, Feagan BG, Martin F, Sutherland LR, Thomson ABR, Williams CN, Nilsson LG, Persson T and the Canadian Inflammatory Bowel Disease Study Group. Oral budesonide for active Crohn's disease. *N Engl J Med* 1994; 331: 836-41.
36. Rutgeerts P, Löfberg R, Malchow H, Lamers C, Olaison G, Jewell D, Danielsson Å, Goebell H, Østergaard-Thomsen O, Lorenz-Meyer H, Hodgson H, Persson T, Seidegård C. A comparison of budesonide with prednisolone for active Crohn's disease. *N Engl J Med* 1994; 331: 842-5.
37. Campieri C, Ferguson A, Doe W and the International Budesonide Study Group. Oral budesonide competes favourably with prednisolone in active Crohn's disease. *Gastroenterology* 1995; 108: A790.
38. Gross V, Andus T, Caesar I, Manns M, Lochs H, Genser D, Schulz J, Bär U, Uberschaer B, Weber A, Gierend M, Ewe K, Schölmerich J. Oral PH-modified release budesonide vs 6-methyl prednisolone in active Crohn's disease. *Gastroenterology* 1995; 108: A828.
39. Löfberg R, Rutgeerts P, Malchow H, Lamers C, Danielsson Å, Olaison G, Jewell D, Østergaard-Thomsen O, Lorenz-Meyer H, Goebell H, Hodgson H, Persson T, Seidegård C. Budesonide prolongs time to relapse in ileal and ileocecal Crohn's disease. A placebo-controlled one year study. *Gut* 1996; 39: 82-6.
40. Greenberg G, Feagan B, Martin F, Sutherland LR, Thomson ABR, Williams CN, Nilsson LG, Persson T and the Canadian Inflammatory Bowel Disease Study Group. Oral budesonide as maintenance treatment for Crohn's disease: a placebo-controlled, dose-ranging study. *Gastroenterology* 1996; 110: 45-51.
41. Ursing B, Alm T, Barany F, Bergelin I, Ganrot-Norlin K, Hoevels J, Huitfeldt B, Jarnerot G, Krause U, Krook A, Lindstrom B, Nordle O, Rosen A. A comparative study of metronidazole and sulfasalazine for active Crohn's disease: the Cooperative Crohn's Disease Study in Sweden. II. Result. *Gastroenterology* 1982; 83: 550-62.
42. Sutherland L, Singleton J, Sessions J, Hanauer SB, Krawitt E, Rankin G, Summers R, Mekhjian H, Greenberger N, Kelly M, Levine J, Thomson A, Alpert E, Prokipchuk E. Double-blind, placebo-controlled trial of metronidazole in Crohn's disease. *Gut* 1991; 32: 1071-5.
43. Bernstein LH, Frank MS, Brandt LJ, Boley SJ. Healing of perineal Crohn's disease with metronidazole. *Gastroenterology* 1980; 79: 357-65.
44. Rutgeerts P, Hiele M, Geboes K, Peeters M, Penninckx F, Aerts R, Kerremans R. Controlled trial of metronidazole treatment for prevention of Crohn's recurrence after ileal resection. *Gastroenterology* 1995; 108: 1617-21.

45. Solomon MJ, McLeod RS, O'Connor BI, Steinhart AH, Greenberg GR, Cohen Z. Combination ciprofloxacin and metronidazole in severe perianal Crohn's disease. *Can J Gastroenterol* 1993; 7: 571-3.
46. Prantera C, Zannoni F, Scribano ML, Berto E, Andreoli A, Kohn A, Luzi C. An antibiotic regimen for the treatment of active Crohn's disease: a randomized controlled clinical trial of metronidazole plus ciprofloxacin. *Am J Gastroenterol* 1996; 91: 328-32.
47. Graham DY, Al-Assi MT, Robinson M. Prolonged remission in Crohn's disease following therapy for Mycobacterium paratuberculosis. *Gastroenterology* 1995; 108: A826.

Recent advances
in gastrointestinal surgery

Gastroesophageal reflux disease and esophageal motility disorders

L. Lundell

Department of Surgery, Sahlgren's University Hospital, University of Gothenburg, Gothenburg, Sweden

Summary

Gastroesophageal reflux disease is a common disorder with a seemingly increasing incidence in the Western countries. Profound acid inhibition therapy has occupied a central role in the medical management of reflux disease both in the short- and long-term perspective. The indications for long-term medical management are fairly similar to that for antireflux surgery. Today the laparoscopic approach to antireflux surgery is totally dominating with promising short-term clinical results. Relapses and failures usually occur early after « conventional-open » antireflux surgery, so it is assumed that the long-term outcome also after laparoscopic antireflux procedures can be expected to be favourable. The motor disorder of the esophagus and gastroesophageal junction which engages the surgeons is primarily achalasia. Achalasia is manometrically characterised by a lack of coordinated peristaltic motor function in the body of the esophagus and a high tone of the lower esophageal sphincter with an incomplete lack of relaxation on swallowing. More seldomly diffuse spasm and nut-crackers esophagus is diagnosed. The laparoscopic-thoracoscopic approaches to these conditions are now quite dominating as the surgical therapeutic option.

Gastroesophageal reflux disease

Recent advances in the medical treatment of gastroesophageal reflux disease now allow the physician to both heal acute episodes of esophagitis and maintain these patients in clinical remission [1-3]. It is also generally accepted that medical therapy can be used as a long-term maintenance therapy and may also be a legitimate alternative to surgery for the management of severe, long-standing gastroesophageal reflux disease [3]. A comprehensive comparison of the true merits of the different treatment options requires, however, generally accepted criteria for the assessment of the severity of the disease with respect both to symptoms and/or the presence of complications. In the medical literature there is a general agreement on the design of studies to be used in clinical science, allowing the assessment of treatment outcomes (such as endoscopic healing and symptom relief) which forms the basis of an objective comparison between different drug regimens. A corresponding consensus on the design of clinical trials over the efficacy of antireflux surgery is unfortunately not available. Despite these methodological obstacles, it can be concluded that the indications for long-term medical as well as for surgical therapy are quite similar [3-10].

Antireflux surgery is designed to improve the function of the gastroesophageal junction and to provide the gastroesophageal reflux patients complete relief of all symptoms and complications of the disease all which occur secondary to deficiencies in the reflux preventing barrier located in the gastroesophageal junction. Ideally, reconstruction of the physiology of the gastroesophageal junction should also permit the patient to swallow normally, belch to relieve distension but hardly to vomit [11-13]. A major effect of fundoplication operations has been shown to be a substantial reduction in the number of transient lower esophageal sphincter relaxations [13]. In addition, the proportion of these relaxations accompanied by reflux is decreased as well as a concomitant increase in the residual pressure at the gastroesophageal junction during sphincter relaxation. This is probably another additional important mechanism to prevent reflux, especially in cases with severe complications of the disease. Previous data have repeatedly shown that fundoplication operations restrain the lower esophageal sphincter relaxation during water swallows by what seems to be a purely mechanical effect [14]. The prevention of reflux during complete lower esophageal sphincter relaxation, even after a fundoplication, suggests that there are other effects of fundoplication on sphincter function separate from that of a single external cuff.

Fundoplications have, since the discovery by Nissen [15] that a fundic wrap prevents reflux, become the most widely used form of antireflux surgery and the efficacy has been established by clinical and endoscopic follow-up and also by esophageal 24 hour pH-monitoring [16-21]. Over the last 3 decades, a number of modifications of the original fundoplication operation have evolved but not every surgeon using the actual technique is as satisfied with the clinical outcome as the originator. Gastroesophageal reflux disease is such a common condition [22, 23] that it is impossible for every patient to be attended by an expert and this might be one important reason for some of the poor results [24, 25]. It is clear that the overwhelming majority of studies report good to excellent results in the order of 80 % or better. By compiling data from controlled, clinical trials, it can be concluded that obvious clinical differences in the efficacy between different antireflux procedures seem not to be prevailing when the outcome is judged with regard to the cumulative reflux relapse rate *(Table I)* [18, 26-32]. Excellent control of reflux symptoms can be obtained with a total fundic wrap, a 270° fundoplication, 180° fundoplication or Hill posterior gastropexi provided that each operation involves a reduction of hiatal hernia coupled with the construction of the valve mechanisms to re-establish gastroesophageal competence. It must be emphasised that these success rates can and should be achieved concomitant with almost zero mortality and morbidity. The problem is, however, that published results usually represent the best results in the field of antireflux surgery and the local level of expertise, at each individual hospital, can vary considerably.

Accordingly, it is reasonable to propose that antireflux surgery should be performed only in centres, where the expertise has been assembled in the management of gastroesophageal reflux disease as well as in the essential diagnostic facilities. Data are now accumulating to show that the short-term outcome after laparoscopic fundoplication is as advantageous as that following open surgery [18, 20]. Long-term follow-up data after laparoscopic procedures are, however, still warranted. A technique that largely eliminates the inter surgeon variation in technique is the introduction of the Angelchik prosthesis. This operations has been shown to be an effective operation in controlling reflux. In controlled, clinical trials presented so far this procedure has been shown to be as effective as Nissen fundoplication in preventing reflux symptoms (see *Table I*). The disadvantages with the prosthesis are the risk of dysphagia and migration of the prosthesis [33]. Consequently this technique is not to be recommended. It should always be born in mind that adequate and sustained reflux control can essentially always be accomplished by an experienced surgeon taking the advantage of wrapping the mobile gastric fundus round the distal esophagus.

Unless there is a clear indication for a thoracic approach, the choice of the abdominal route is to be preferred. The thoracic procedure takes twice as long to accomplish as a transabdominal fundoplication and major postoperative problems seem to be more frequent and are specific for the repair such as post-thoracotomy pain.

Table I. The clinical outcome of different antireflux procedures when evaluated in prospective, controlled, randomised clinical trials.

References	Follow-up period	Procedure	Excellent to good results (%)	Failure rate (%)
Washer et al. (1984)	5 years	Nissen (360º)	65	20
		Roux-en-Y	91	41
De Meester et al. (1974)	30-696 days	Hill	47	53
		Nissen (360º)	100	0
		Belsey (270º)	80	20
Gear et al. (1984)	1-2 years	Angelchik	96	4
		Nissen (360º)	81	19
Stuart et al. (1989)	38 months	Angelchik	77	23
		Nissen (360º)	94	6
Hill et al. (1994)	7 years	Angelchik	77	23
		Nissen-Rossetti (360º)	88	8
Kmiot et al. (1991)	3-24 months	Angelchik	60-72	28
		Nissen	85-88	12
Thor, Silander (1989)	5 years	Nissen (360º)	67	25
		Toupet (180-200º)	95	0
Lundell et al. (1991)	6 months	Nissen-Rossetti (360º)	95	3
		Toupet (180-200º)	95	3
Walther et al. (1992)	13 months	Nissen (360º)	92	8
		Lind (300º)	96	4
Janssen et al. (1993)	12 months	Nissen (360º)	90	0
		Lig. teres gastropexi	40	60
Lundell et al. (1996)	> 3 years	Nissen-Rossetti (360º)	4	11
		Toupet (180-200º)	6	6

Although antireflux surgery is generally very effective in controlling gastroesophageal reflux, some failures are proven unavoidable [34-40]. The frequency by which these postfundoplication symptoms have been reported varies considerably between series. Dysphagia is frequently reported during the early postoperative period but vanishes with the passage of time. Some clinical studies even report an impressive number of patients being able to vomit postoperatively, especially when interviewed after many years. Similar clinical information should, however, cause concern regarding an eventual disruption of the wrap rather than an example of subsidence of complaints with the passage of time. A number of technical considerations have been focused on and alleged to counteract some of these postfundoplication problems but it must be concluded, based on data from controlled, randomised clinical trials, that as yet no significant differences with regard to postfundoplication symptoms have been firmly established among different antireflux procedures. There is a wide spread consensus, however, among experienced surgeons, that when a complete (360° wrap) is done it has to be both floppy and short, which means that the gastric fundus has to be widely mobilised and that the fundoplication done about 1 cm long. However, a clear tendency has been reported in some trials that partial fundoplication procedures seem to be associated with less troublesome postfundoplication complaints [28, 31].

Primary esophageal motor disorders

Abnormalities in the motor function of the esophageal body and/or the lower esophageal sphincter can give rise to a number of disorders that usually result in dysphagia and/or regurgitation [41-43]. These symptoms may be due to a non-relaxing lower esophageal sphincter, disorganised contractions of the esophageal body or a combination of both. With the introduction of esophageal manometry, a number of primary esophageal motility disorders have been classified as separate disease entities. These include achalasia, diffuse esophageal spasm, nutcracker esophagus and the hypertensive lower esophageal sphincter *(Table II)*. The classification of these disorders is usually based on analysis of the manometry recordings of only a few water swallows performed in a laboratory setting but the recently introduced technique of ambulatory 24 hour monitoring [44] of esophageal motor activity multiplies the number of esophageal contractions available for analysis and provides an opportunity to assess esophageal motor function under a variety of physiological situations [45].

Achalasia

Dysphagia is a primary symptom of esophageal motor disorders. Its perception by the patient is a balance between the severity of the underlying abnormality and the adjustment made by the patient in altering his or her eating habits. Because the adjustment is initially unconscious, detailed questioning is required to uncover its extent. It is also important to distinguish vomiting from regurgitation, because the patient may mislead the clinician by describing the regurgitation of blunt tasting, recently ingested food, as vomiting. In addition, a history of weight loss should be sought. These assessments help to quantitate the dysphagia and provide a measure of the extent to which the disorder has interfered with the patients physical and social health.

The aim of treatment of achalasia is to improve symptoms and restore transit of saliva and food by reducing the resistance of the lower esophageal sphincter. The recent development of laparoscopic surgery has renewed the interest in the surgical therapy of achalasia [46-55]. A crucial point in the myotomy technique is the extension of the myotomy into the stomach and also to include the entire sphincter in the myotomy. Incompleteness leads to persistent or recurrent achalasia. The changing direction of the muscular fibres from circular in the esophagus to oblique in the cardia are important land marks. It has been shown that a partial fundoplication added to the myotomy can have obvious clinical advantages in controlling the reflux that most likely occurs in a great majority of cases after adequate myotomy.

Table II. Manometric criteria of primary motor disorders of the esophagus.

	Manometry
Achalasia	Incomplete LES relaxation Aperistalsis High basal LES tone
Diffuse esophageal spasm	Simultaneous (non peristaltic) contractions Intermittent normal peristalsis Multipeaked contractions Increased amplitude and duration
« Nutcracker » esophagus	Mean peristaltic amplitude >180 mm Hg in the distal esophagus Normal peristaltic sequence
Hypertensive LES	High basal tone (> 26 mm Hg?) Normal relaxation Normal peristalsis

It is generally agreed that the drug treatment of achalasia is ineffective. The only treatment of widespread use is surgical myotomy, balloon dilatation and more recently botulinum toxin injection [56]. Only one randomised trial [49] has compared myotomy with dilatation and this showed a clear advantage of myotomy combined with an antireflux procedure.

Four important principles have to be followed when surgical myotomy of the lower esophageal sphincter is performed: (1) minimal dissection of the cardia, (2) adequate distal myotomy to reduce outflow resistance, (3) prevention of postoperative reflux and (4) prevention of rehealing of the myotomy site. These principles are followed regardless of whether the myotomy is performed thoracoscopically, or through the abdomen. Postoperatively almost all patients experience immediate improvement in dysphagia.

Follow-up data from laparoscopic myotomy with or without antireflux procedure as well as after thoracoscopic myotomy is most reassuring. Greater and longer experiences are, however, needed in order to have a comprehensive view on the true clinical durability of these therapeutic effects.

Diffuse and segmental esophageal spasm

This motor disorder is characterised clinically by substernal chest-pain and/or dysphagia. Diffuse esophageal spasm differs from classic achalasia in that it is primarily a disease of the esophageal body, it produces a less degree of dysphagia, it causes chest-pain and has less effect on the patient general condition. True diffuse spasm is a rare condition, occurring approximately five times less frequently than achalasia [45, 57, 58]. Manometric abnormalities may be present in the total length of the esophageal body but are usually confined to the distal two thirds. In segmental spasm the manometric abnormalities are confined to a short segment of the esophagus. The classic manometric finding of these patients is the frequent occurrence of simultaneous and repetitive esophageal contractions with abnormally high amplitude and long duration.

The lower esophageal sphincter in these patients usually shows normal resting pressure and relaxation on swallowing. A hypertensive sphincter with poor relaxation may, however, also rarely be present. In patients with advanced disease, the radiographic appearance has labelled the term « corkscrew esophagus » or « pseudodiverticulosis ». Patients with segmental or diffuse esophageal spasm can also compartmentalise the esophagus and develop an epiphrenic or mid-esophageal diverticulum.

A long esophageal myotomy is indicated for dysphagia caused by any motor disorder characterised by segmental and generalised simultaneous contraction in a patient whose symptoms are not relieved by medical therapy [42, 43, 50, 59]. The myotomy will abolish the simultaneous waves, leading to an improvement if these waves were responsible for the chest-pain and dysphagia. It has been suggested that if the ambulatory motility monitoring shows that more than 70 % of the waves are simultaneous, the loss of the few remaining peristaltic waves is likely to be counterbalanced by the beneficial abolition of simultaneous waves. This might shift the balance in favour of myotomy. Patients whose only symptom is chest-pain do not, as frequently, have a good result after surgical myotomy. The myotomy should ideally extend distally partly across the lower esophageal sphincter because the resistance of a normal lower esophageal sphincter may still be too great for the myotomised esophageal body to overcome. The technique of long esophageal myotomy is essentially the same as for myotomy of the lower esophageal sphincter. These operations are done by use of minimal invasive techniques, applying thoracoscopic approaches. This surgical technique nowadays also allows concomitant resection of distal and mid-esophageal diverticuli.

Previous published series report between 40 and 92 % symptomatic improvement but interpretation is difficult because of the small number of patients involved and the varying criteria for diagnosis of the primary motor abnormality. When this is accurately done, 93 % of the patients had effective palliation of dysphagia after a mean follow-up time of 5 years and 89 % would have the procedure again if it was necessary.

References

1. Bell JIV, Hunt RH. Role of gastric acid suppression in the treatment of gastroesophageal reflux disease. *Gut* 1992; 33: 118-24.
2. Bell NJV, Burget D, Howden CW, Wilkinson J, Hunt RH. Appropriate acid suppression for the management of gastroesophageal reflux disease. *Digestion* 1992; 51 (suppl. 1): 59-67.
3. Lundell L. Acid suppression in the long-term treatment of peptic stricture and Barrett's esophagus. *Digestion* 1992; 51 (Suppl. 1): 49-58.
4. Armstrong D, Nicolet M, Monnier T, et al. Maintenance therapy: is there still a place for antireflux surgery? *World J Surg* 1992; 6: 300.
5. Behar J, Sheahan DG, Biancani P, Spiro HM, Storer EH. Medical and surgical management of reflux esophagitis. A 38-month report on a prospective clinical trial. *N Engl J Med* 1975; 293: 263-8.
6. DeMeester TR, Johnson LF, Kent AH. Evaluation of current operations for the prevention of gastroesophageal reflux. *Ann Surg* 1974; 180: 511.
7. Dent J, Yeomans ND. Acid related diseases: improving the treatment options. *Digestion* 1992; 51: Suppl. 1.
8. Feussner H, Petri A, Walker S. et al. The modified AFP-score: an attempt to make the results of antireflux surgery comparable. *Br J Surg* 1991; 78: 942.
9. Jamieson GG, Duranceau AC, Deschamps, C. Surgical treatment of gastroesophageal reflux disease. In: Jamieson GG, Duranceau AC, eds. *Gastresophageal reflux*. Philadelphia: WB Saunders, 1988; chapt. 10.
10. Spechler JS, et al. Comparison of medical and surgical therapy for complicated gastroesophageal reflux disease in veterans. *N Engl J Med* 1992; 326: 786.
11. Bancewicz J, Mughal M, Marples M. The lower esophageal sphincter after floppy Nissen fundoplication. *Br J Surg* 1987; 74: 162.
12. DeMeester TR, Stein HJ. Minimizing the side effects of antireflux surgery. *World J Surg* 1992; 16: 335.
13. Ireland AC, Holloway RH, Toouli J, Dent J. Mechanisms underlying the antireflux action of fundoplication. *Gut* 1993; 34: 303.
14. Little AG. Mechanism of action of antireflux surgery: theory and facts. *World J Surg* 1992; 16; 320.
15. Nissen R. Eine einfache Operation zur Be-einflussung der Refluxosophagitis. *Schw Med Wochenschr* 1956; 86: 590.
16. Negre SB, Markkula HT, Keyrilainen O, Matikainen M. Nissen fundoplication. *Am J Surg* 1983; 146: 635.
17. Rossetti N, Hell K. Fundoplication for treatment of gastroesophageal reflux disease in hiatal hernia. *World J Surg* 1977; 1: 439.
18. Cadière GB, Houben JJ, Bruyns J, Himpens J, Panser JM, Gelin M. Laparoscopic Nissen fundoplication: technique and preliminary results. *Br J Surg* 1994; 81: 400-3.
19. DeMeester TR, Bonavina L, Albertucci M. Nissen fundoplication for gastroesophageal reflux disease. Evaluation of primary repair in 100 consecutive patients. *Ann Surg* 1986; 204: 9.
20. Jamieson GG, Watson DL, Britten-Jones R, Mitchell PC, Anvari M. Laparoscopic Nissen fundoplication. *Ann Surg* 1984; 2: 137-45.
21. Johansson J, Johnson F, Joelsson BE, Florén CH, Walther, B. Outcome from 5 years after 360° fundoplication for gastroesophageal reflux disease. *Br J Surg* 1993; 80: 46.
22. Weinbeck M, Barnert J. Epidemiology of reflux disease and reflux esophagitis. *Scand J Gastroenterol* 1989; 24 (Suppl.) 156: 7-13.
23. Heading RC. Epidemiology of esophageal reflux disease. *Scand J Gastroenterol* 1989; 24 (suppl. 168): 33.
24. Donahue PE, Schiesinger PK, Sluss KF, et al. Esophagocardiomyotomy- floppy Nissen fundoplication effectively treats achalasia without causing esophageal obstruction. *Surgery* 1994; 116: 719-25.

25. Donahue PE, Samuelson S, Nyhus LM, Bombeck CT. The floppy Nissen fundoplication. *Arch Surg* 1985; 120: 663.
26. Gear MWL, Gillison EW, Dowling BL. Randomised prospective trial of the Angelchik antireflux prosthesis. *Br J Surg* 1984; 71: 681.
27. Kimiot WA, Kirby RM, Akinola D, Temple G. Prospective randomised trial of Nissen fundoplication and Angelchik prosthesis in the surgical treatment of medically refractory gastroesophageal reflux disease. *Br J Surg* 1991; 78: 1181.
28. Lundell L, Abrahamsson H, Ruth M, Sandberg N, Olbe L. Lower esophageal sphincter characteristics and esophageal acid exposure following partial or 360° fundoplication: results of a prospective, randomized, clinical study. *World J Surg* 1991; 15: 115.
29. Stuart RC, Dawson K, Keeling P, Byrne PJ, Hennessy TPJ. A prospective randomized trial of Angelchik prosthesis versus Nissen fundoplication. *Br J Surg* 1989; 76: 86.
30. Thor KBA, Silander T. A long-term randomized prospective trial of the Nissen procedure versus a modified Toupet technique. *Ann Surg* 1989; 210: 719.
31. Walker SJ, Holt S, Sanderson CJ, Stoddard CJ. Comparison of Nissen total and Lind partial transabdominal fundoplication in the treatment of gastroesophageal reflux. *Br J Surg* 1992; 79: 410.
32. Washer BF, Gear MWL, Dowling BL, *et al.* Randomised prospective trial of Roux-en-Y duodenal diversion vs fundoplication for severe reflux esophagitis. *Br J Surg* 1984; 71: 181.
33. Durrans D, Armstrong CP, Taylor TV. The Angelchik anti-reflux prosthesis - some reservations. *Br J Surg* 1985; 72: 525.
34. Hill LD, Lives R, Stevenson JK, Pearson JM. Reoperation for disruption and recurrence after Nissen fundoplication. *Arch Surg* 1979; 114: 542.
35. Garstin WI, Hohnston GW, Kennedy TL, Spencer ES. Nissen fundoplication: the unhappy 15 %. *J R Coll Surg*, Edinburgh, 1986; 31: 207.
36. Leonardi HK, Corzier RE, Elils FH. Reoperation for complications of the Nissen fundoplication. *J Thorac Cardiovasc Surg* 1989; 81: 50.
37. Maher JW, Hocking MP, Woodward ER. Reoperations for esophagitis following failed antireflux procedures. *Ann Surg* 1985; 201: 723.
38. Negre JB. Post-fundoplication symptoms. Do they restrict the success of Nissen fundoplication? *Ann Surg* 1983; 198: 698.
39. Siewert RJ, Isolauri J, Feussner H. Reoperation following failed fundoplication. *World J Surg* 1989; 13: 791.
40. Skinner DB. Surgical management after failed antireflux operations. *World J Surg* 1992; 16: 359.
41. Castell DO, Richter JE, Dalton CB, eds. *Esophageal motility testing.* New York: Elsevier, 1987.
42. DeMeester TR, Stein HJ. Surgery for esophageal motor disorders. In: Castell DO, ed. *The Esophagus.* Boston: Little Brown 1992; 401-39.
43. DeMeester TR. Surgery for esophageal motor disorders. *Ann Thorac Surg* 1982; 34: 225.
44. Stein HJ, DeMeester TR, Eypasch EP. Ambulatory 24-hour esophageal manometry in the evaluation of esophageal motor disorders and non-cardiac chest pain. *Surgery* 1991; 110: 753-63.
45. Eypasch EP, Stein HJ, DeMeester TR, *et al.* A new technique to define and clarify esophageal motor disorders. *Am J Surg* 1990; 59: 144.
46. Avranitakis C. Achalasia of the esophagus: a reappraisal of esophagomyotomy vs forceful pneumatic dilatation. *Dig Dis Sci* 1975; 20: 841-6.
47. Andreollo NA, Earlam RJ. Heller's myotomy for achalasia: is an added antireflux procedure necessary? *Br J Surg* 1987; 74: 765-9.
48. Bonavina L, Nosadinia A, Bardini R, *et al.* Primary treatment of esophageal achalasia: long-term results of myotomy and Dor fundoplication. *Arch Surg* 1992; 127: 222-6.
49. Csendes A, Braghetto I, Henriquez A, *et al.* Late results of a prospective randomised study comparing forceful dilatation and oesophagomyotomy in patients with achalasia. *Gut* 1989; 30: 299-304.

50. Cuschieri A. Endoscopic esophageal myotomy for specific motility disorders and non cardiac chest pain. *Endosc Surg Allied Technol* 1993; 1: 280-7.
51. Eckardt VF, Aignherr C, Bernhard G. Predictors of outcome in patients with achalasia treated by pneumatic dilation. *Gastroenterology* 1992; 103: 1732-8.
52. Jara FM, Toledo-Pereya LH, Lewis JW, *et al.* Long-term results of esophagomyotomy for achalasia of esophagus. *Arch Surg* 1979; 114: 935-6.
53. Okike N, Payne WS. Esophagomyotomy versus forceful dilation for achalasia of the esophagus: results in 899 patients. *Ann Thorac Surg* 1979; 23: 119.
54. Paricio P, Martinez de Haro L, Ortiz A, *et al.* Achalasia of the cardia: long-term results of oesophagomyotomy and posterior partial fundoplication. *Br J Surg* 1990; 77: 1371-4.
55. Pellegrini C, Leichter R, Patti M, *et al.* Thoracoscopic esophageal myotomy in the treatment of achalasia. *Ann Thorac Surg* 1992; 56: 680-2.
56. Pasricha PJ, Ravich WJ, Hendrix TR, *et al.* Intrasphincteric botulinum toxin for the treatment of achalasia. *N Engl J Med* 1995; 332: 774-8.
57. Eypasch E, DeMeester TR, Klingman R, *et al.* Physiological assessment and surgical management of diffuse esophageal spasm. *J Thorac Cardiovasc Surg* 1992; 104: 859-68.
58. Gillies M, Nicks R, Skyring A. Clinical, manometric, and pathological studies in diffuse oesophageal spasm. *Br Med J* 1967; 2: 527.
59. Pellegrini C, Wetter LA, Patti M, *et al.* Thoracoscopic esophagomyotomy. *Ann Surg* 1992; 216: 291.

Adjuvant therapy and surgery of esophageal cancer

L. Bonavina, A. Peracchia

Department of General and Oncologic Surgery, University of Milan, Ospedale Maggiore Policlinico, IRCCS, Milano, Italy

Summary

Surgical resection is still the mainstay of treatment for esophageal cancer, but the prognosis continues to be unsatisfactory in tumors extending beyond the mucosa and in those accompanied by nodal metastases. The proposal to use preoperative neo-adjuvant therapy began when it became evident that most patients develop systemic metastases without local recurrence, and that postoperative adjuvant therapy is largely ineffective. A variety of neoadjuvant approaches have been investigated in an effort to induce down-staging of the tumor, increase the resectability of the tumor at unfavorable locations, eliminate potential systemic micrometastases, and ultimately to prolong survival. Although preoperative chemoradiation pilot studies provide the most encouraging results to date, both in patients with potentially resectable and in those with locally advanced esophageal tumors, it should be remembered that these are non-randomized, non-controlled studies, and the definitive determination of benefit must await the final results of prospective trials. Postoperative adjuvant therapy seems to play a role in the context of a sequential multimodality treatment which should include neoadjuvant regimens.

Advances in surgical technique and perioperative management have made esophageal resection an operation of acceptable risk [1, 2]. However, despite the efforts to achieve a curative (R0) resection [3-8], the overall prognosis of patients with esophageal carcinoma has not improved for the following reasons: (1) the tumor extends through the esophageal wall in the majority of patients at the time of presentation; (2) systemic metastases occur early in the course of the disease; and, (3) radicality is technically impossible in tumors located at or above the level of the carina because of the close anatomical relationship with the tracheo-bronchial tree [9, 10]. Surgery alone allows favorable cure rates only in patients with early stage esophageal carcinoma [11]. Unfortunately, most patients presenting with symptomatic esophageal carcinoma in Western countries have T3-T4 tumors and/or nodal metastases. This represents the rationale for the use of neoadjuvant (pre-operative) therapy [12]. A variety of neo-adjuvant approaches have been investigated in an effort to induce down-staging of the tumor, increase the resectability of the tumor at unfavorable locations, eliminate potential systemic micrometastases, identify the patients who might benefit from further postoperative chemotherapy, and ultimately improve disease-free and overall survival [13]. The combination of chemotherapy and concurrent radiation has been advocated based on the fact that these two therapeutic modalities may have independent activity against different tumor cell subpopulations and cells that are resistant to one modality may be sensitive to the other [14].

Selection of patients for neoadjuvant therapy

Stage of tumor

According to the TNM staging system, curative (R0) resection means absence of residual tumor after treatment in any of the margins of the specimen (proximal, distal, and lateral margin). It has been shown that a R0 resection is the major independent prognostic factor in patients with esophageal carcinoma [15]. A R0 resection can be anticipated with a high degree of certainty in patients who have a tumor confined within the esophageal wall on endoscopic ultrasonography. These patients should be submitted to primary surgery. In contrast, a R0 resection is unlikely if endoscopic ultrasonography shows wall penetration or if the stenosis cannot be passed with the instrument, particularly if the tumor is located at or above the level of the carina. In these patients, the results of primary surgical therapy are dismal and neoadjuvant therapy should be considered if the patient is fit for subsequent surgical resection. More recently, laparoscopy and laparoscopic ultrasonography have been proposed to further increase accuracy of staging [16, 17].

Physiological patient status

Combined modality therapy should only be considered in patients with adequate performance status (> 2 WHO) and pulmonary, cardiac, renal, hepatic and hemopoietic reserve. Forced expiratory volume in 1 second (FEV1) and ejection fraction are the best indicators of cardiopulmonary reserve [1]. Patient's cooperation is another major parameter to be considered before entering a neoadjuvant program.

Histological tumor type

There has been a significant increase in the prevalence of adenocarcinoma of the esophagus in recent years [18]. Neoadjuvant therapy in patients with potentially resectable adenocarcinoma of the esophagus is still investigational. Preliminary results of non-randomized trials show a complete histopathologic response in up to 20 % of patients [19-21]. A combined modality approach can be of benefit in patients with locally advanced esophageal carcinoma irrespective of the histological type, but the choice of the regimen should be adapted to the tumor type [13].

Results of neoadjuvant therapy for potentially resectable carcinoma

Preoperative radiotherapy

The use of preoperative radiotherapy has been extensively evaluated in phase II and phase III trials. All randomized studies have failed to demonstrate an increased resection rate or increased survival in patients receiving preoperative radiotherapy as compared to those treated by primary surgery. The only benefit appeared to be an improvement in local tumor control. As a consequence, neoadjuvant radiotherapy alone has been abandoned [22, 23].

Preoperative chemotherapy

The majority of studies on preoperative chemotherapy in patients with potentially resectable tumor have been non-random phase II trials. Two or more cycles of cisplatin-based combination chemotherapy are used, commonly associated to 5-fluorouracil. A typical dose schedule is: cisplatin 100 mg/m^2 (either given entirely on day 1 or in divided doses on days 1-5) and 5-fluorouracil 600-1000 mg/m^2 given as continuous 24-hour infusion on days 1-5. The cycle is repeated at 3 weeks and 6 weeks, and surgery is performed 3 weeks after completion of the last cycle. Major side-effects include mucositis, diarrhea, and myelosuppression. With adequate hydration, significant renal dysfunction is seen in less than 5 % of the patients. When the results of the trials are taken together, it appears that chemotherapy does not increase postoperative morbidity and mortality. A clinical response, complete or partial, can be seen in up to 70 % of patients, while a complete histopathological response is rare. Compared to primary surgical resection, preoperative chemotherapy does not increase the resection rate, rate of R0 resections, or median survival. A survival advantage appears to exist only in patients manifesting a major objective response to preoperative therapy [12, 13].

Preoperative chemoradiotherapy

The very low rate of complete histopathologic response with preoperative chemotherapy prompted several investigators to assess the combination of preoperative chemoradiotherapy. The results of phase II trials indicate a marked increase in complete histopathologic response rate (20-40 %) at the expense of increased postoperative morbidity and mortality. Therefore, this therapeutic regimen remains investigational and should not be used outside the context of clinical trials [12, 13].

Results of neoadjuvant therapy for locally advanced carcinoma

The experience with combined modality therapy in this subgroup of patients is limited. No prospective trials exist, and the majority of phase II studies have been published in an abstract form only. Generally, neoadjuvant therapy has lead to down-staging of the primary tumor in a substantial proportion of patients, increased rate of R0 resections, and prolonged survival compared to historical controls [24]. Combined chemoradiotherapy is more effective than chemotherapy alone, but the higher response rate is achieved at the expense of a higher morbidity and mortality rate. Patients who show a complete histopathologic response after chemoradiotherapy have a clear survival benefit. First-line chemoradiation followed by surgery is feasible in dedicated centers, but care must be taken to keep morbidity and mortality low. The optimal sequence in this multimodality approach is presently unknown [12].

Prediction of response to neoadjuvant therapy

Histopathologic response to neoadjuvant therapy cannot be reliably predicted based on clinical response. Residual tumor is often found in the resected specimen in patients who had complete clinical response; conversely, up to 10 % of patients with partial or no clinical response may have a complete histopathologic response. The identification of p53 mutations in cell cultured from endoscopic biopsies [25] and *in vitro* preoperative chemosensitivity testing [26] may help in the future to tailor the neoadjuvant regimen to the individual patient.

Assessment of response after neoadjuvant therapy

Evaluation of response is the critical issue in determining the effectiveness of a neoadjuvant regimen and planning subsequent therapy. However, clinical assessment of tumor response is difficult and no reliable criteria exist. Negative biopsies at post-treatment endoscopy do not guarantee complete histopathologic response; in about one third of these patients, viable neoplastic cells can be detected in the muscularis propria or lymph nodes even when the mucosa appears completely healed. Endoscopic ultrasonography has proven inaccurate in assessing the T parameter. The major drawback of the currently available imaging techniques is the difficulty in distinguishing residual tumor from fibrotic tissue [27]. As clinical restaging after neoadjuvant treatment is often inaccurate, one must be very cautious when deciding to exclude a patient from surgery.

Role of primary chemoradiotherapy without surgery

The role of surgery after neoadjuvant therapy has been questioned due to the impressive rate of response with chemoradiotherapy and the potentially increased risk of resection in these patients. However, local tumor recurrences are common in patients undergoing chemoradiation alone, underlying the essential role of surgical resection after neoadjuvant therapy [28, 29]. In patients who are not surgical candidates because of high operative risk or residual disease, concurrent chemotherapy and radiotherapy given as definitive treatment is more effective than radiation therapy alone [30]. To date, little information exists regarding the feasibility and effectiveness of salvage surgery following high dose radiotherapy (> 50 Gy) [12].

Role of postoperative regimens

Adjuvant therapy

There is no consensus on the need of postoperative therapy in patients with no residual disease, *i.e.* R0 resection. Even in the absence of nodal metastases, transmural tumors have a poor prognosis. Adjuvant radiation therapy may decrease the incidence of local recurrences, but has no impact on survival [31]. There are no randomized studies investigating the effects of adjuvant chemotherapy. This therapeutic modality seems mostly indicated in patients who have already responded well to preoperative chemotherapy [12].

Additive therapy

Some form of postoperative therapy should theoretically be given to control residual disease left behind by the surgeon, *i.e.* R1-R2 resections. However, there is no proof that such additive treatment is effective. Chemoradiation therapy is reasonable in patients with residual disease at or above the level of the carina, otherwise it can be postponed until the recurrence will become clinically evident. In the presence of gross residual disease, the chances of cure are very low [12].

Conclusions

Multimodality therapy of esophageal cancer is feasible and safe in selected patients; it should be carried out in specialized units with expertise in both therapeutic endoscopy and esophageal surgery, and ready access to radiotherapy and chemotherapy services.

A survival benefit with neoadjuvant therapy can be expected only in responders; therefore, until the final results of ongoing trials will become available, primary resection remains the therapy of choice. The benefits of neoadjuvant therapy in patients with locally advanced esophageal carcinoma are evident from uncontrolled studies; therefore, first-line chemoradiotherapy is justified in dedicated centers. Surgical resection is essential for local tumor control after chemoradiotherapy. The operation should only be performed in physiologically fit patients when a complete tumor resection can reasonably be anticipated. Adjuvant therapy seems justified in the context of a sequential multimodality approach which should include neoadjuvant chemotherapy or chemoradiotherapy.

References

1. DeMeester T, Barlow A. Surgery and current management for cancer of the esophagus and cardia. *Curr Probl Cancer* 1988; 12: 241-327.
2. Law S, Fok M, Wong J. Risk analysis in resection of squamous cell carcinoma of the esophagus. *World J Surg* 1994; 18: 339-46.
3. Skinner D. En bloc resection for neoplasms of the esophagus and cardia. *J Thorac Cardiovasc Surg* 1983; 85: 59-71.
4. Peracchia A, Bardini R, Castoro C, et al. La lymphadenectomie dans le traitement du cancer de l'œsophage intrathoracique. *Ann Chir* 1990; 44: 9-17.
5. Collard J, Otte J, Reynaert M, Fiasse R, Kestens P. Feasibility and effectiveness of en bloc resection of the esophagus for esophageal cancer. Results of a prospective study. *Int Surg* 1991; 76: 209-13.
6. Lerut T, De Leyn P, Coosemans W, et al. Surgical strategies in esophageal carcinoma with emphasis on radical lymphadenectomy. *Ann Surg* 1992; 216: 583-90.
7. Siewert J, Roder J. Lymphadenectomy in esophageal cancer surgery. *Dis Esoph* 1992; 5: 91-8.
8. Akiyama H, Tsurumaru M, Udagawa H, Kajiama Y. Radical lymph node dissection for cancer of the thoracic esophagus. *Ann Surg* 1994; 220: 364-73.
9. Muller J, Erasmi H, Stelzner M, Zieren U, Pichlmaier H. Surgical therapy of oesophageal carcinoma. *Br J Surg* 1990; 77: 845-77.
10. Kelsen D. Combined modality therapy of esophageal cancer. In: Peracchia A *et al.*, eds. *Recent advances in diseases of the esophagus*. Bologna: Monduzzi, 1996: 413-8.
11. Bonavina L. Early esophageal cancer: results of a European multicenter survey. *Br J Surg* 1995; 82: 98-101.
12. Ruol A, et al. Multimodality treatment for non-metastatic cancer of the thoracic esophagus. *Dis Esoph* 1996, 9 (suppl. 1): 39-55.
13. Fink U, Stein H, Bochtler H, et al. Neoadjuvant therapy for squamous cell esophageal carcinoma. *Ann Oncol* 1994; 5 (suppl. 3): 17-26.
14. Vokes E. Interactions of chemotherapy and radiation. *Semin Oncol* 1993; 20: 70-9.
15. Siewert J, Dittler H. Esophageal carcinoma: impact of staging on treatment. *Endoscopy* 1993; 25: 28-32.
16. Watt I, Stewart I, Anderson D, Bell G, Anderson J. Laparoscopy, ultrasound and computed tomography in cancer of the oesophagus and gastric cardia: a prospective comparison for detecting intra-abdominal metastases. *Br J Surg* 1989; 76: 1036-9.
17. O'Brien M, Fitzgerald E, Lee G, et al. A prospective comparison of laparoscopy and imaging in the staging of esophagogastric cancer before surgery. *Am J Gastroenterol* 1995; 90: 2191-4.
18. Pera M, Cameron A, Trastek V, Carpenter H, Zinsmeister A. Increasing incidence of adenocarcinoma of the esophagus and esophagogastric junction. *Gastroenterology* 1993; 104: 510-3.
19. Wolfe W, Vaughn A, Seigler H, et al. Survival of patients with carcinoma of the esophagus treated with combined-modality therapy. *J Thorac Cardiovasc Surg* 1993; 105: 749-55.
20. Hoff S, Stewart J, Sawyers J, et al. Preliminary results with neoadjuvant therapy and resection for esophageal carcinoma. *Ann Thorac Surg* 1993; 56: 282-6.
21. Hennessy T. Multimodal therapy for carcinoma of the cardia. *Dis Esoph* 1996; 9: 187-90.
22. Gignoux M, Roussel A, Paillot B, et al. The value of preoperative radiotherapy in esophageal cancer: results of a study of the EORTC. *World J Surg* 1987; 11: 426-32.
23. Coia L, Sauter E. Esophageal cancer. *Curr Probl Cancer* 1994; 18: 189-248.
24. Castoro C, Ruol A, Chiarion-Sileni V, et al. *Long-term results of surgery after DDP and 5-FU combination chemotherapy for locally advanced squamous cell esophageal carcinoma*. Proceedings 2nd International conference on biology, prevention and treatment of gastrointestinal malignancies. Koln, Germany, 1995: 199 (Abstract).
25. Saito T, Hikita M, Kohno K, et al. Different sensitivities of human esophageal cancer cells to multiple anti-cancer agents and related mechanisms. *Cancer* 1992; 70: 2402-9.

26. Okuma T, Yoshioka M, Isechi S, *et al.* Preoperative chemotherapy for esophageal cancer based on chemosensitivity testing. *J Thorac Cardiovasc Surg* 1994; 108: 823-9.
27. Rice T, Boyce G, Sivak M, Adelstein D, Kirby T. Esophageal carcinoma: esophageal ultrasound assessment of preoperative chemotherapy. *Ann Thorac Surg* 1992; 53: 972-7.
28. Gil P, Denham J, Jamieson G, *et al.* Patterns of treatment failure and prognostic factors associated with the treatment of esophageal carcinoma with chemotherapy and radiotherapy either as sole treatment or followed by surgery. *J Clin Oncol* 1992; 10: 1037-43.
29. Kavanagh B, Anscher M, Leopold L, *et al.* Patterns of failure following combined modality therapy for esophageal cancer. *Int J Radiat Oncol Biol Phys* 1992; 24: 633-42.
30. Herskovic A, Martz K, Al-Sarraf M, *et al.* Combined chemotherapy and radiotherapy compared with radiotherapy alone in patients with cancer of the esophagus. *N Engl J Med* 1992; 326: 1593-8.
31. Fok M, Sham J, Choy D, Cheng S, Wong J. Postoperative radiotherapy for carcinoma of the esophagus: a prospective randomized controlled study. *Surgery* 1993; 113: 138-47.

Repair of the anal sphincter

M.A. Kamm

St Mark's Hospital, Northwick Park, Watford Road Harrow, Middlesex HA1 3UJ, UK

Summary

Successful anal sphincter surgery for faecal incontinence depends on accurate characterisation of symptoms and sphincter pathology. Anal endosonography has revealed that « neurogenic incontinence » is uncommon, with most patients having structural sphincter damage involving one or both of the internal and external anal sphincter muscles. Post anal repair benefits only a quarter of patients long term. The most common sphincter injury is anterior disruption related to childbirth, and overlap repair is successful in 80 percent of patients. Isolated internal anal sphincter repair is not successful. When simple repair is not feasible, a high pressure zone can be created using gracilis or gluteus striated muscle transposition, with or without chronic electrical stimulation. The results are good for idiopathic incontinence, moderate after abdominoperineal cancer resection, and least good in patients with congenital abnormalities. New alternatives include the artificial sphincter, in which preliminary results are encouraging, and spinal sacral stimulation.

Mechanisms of continence

The preservation of faecal continence is dependent on a structurally and functionally intact anal sphincter mechanism and normal rectal and large bowel function. The internal anal sphincter smooth muscle is responsible for most of the resting pressure within the anal canal, and impaired internal anal sphincter function characteristically results in passive faecal incontinence, that is the loss of bowel contents without the patients awareness (sometimes known as soiling). The striated muscle external anal sphincter is responsible for a small part of the normal resting pressure, but more importantly provides a substantial increase in anal pressure when intra-abdominal or bowel pressure increases. This can be *via* sacral reflexes or *via* voluntary contraction. Impaired external anal sphincter function most commonly results in urge faecal incontinence, that is the inability to consciously suppress defaecation [1, 2]. This symptom specificity for impaired function of a particular muscle is not absolute. Occasionally patients experience both passive and urge incontinence because both muscles are damaged, or because the internal anal sphincter is no longer supported circumferentially by the external anal sphincter ring.

Incontinence can also occur when the anal sphincter is structurally and functionally normal, but the bowel is producing high pressures which the sphincter cannot resist. Such a situation, which results in urge incontinence, can occur in patients with irritable bowel syndrome, inflammatory bowel disease, radiation bowel disease, and infectious diarrhoea. The large bowel is capable of producing contractions which are of a very high amplitude, for example 500 cm of water.

To treat incontinence appropriately requires careful identification of the patient's symptoms, including not only the sphincter abnormality but also the nature of associated bowel function. For example, the results of sphincter repair may be suboptimal in a patient, despite a good anatomical result, if the patient has coexistent irritable bowel syndrome and generates high bowel pressures in association with urgent semiformed stool.

Sphincter trauma

Childbirth is the commonest cause of anal sphincter damage. Thirteen percent of women having their first vaginal delivery develop new bowel symptoms of incontinence or urgency. A third of all first vaginal deliveries are associated with structural changes demonstrable by anal endosonography [3]. The commonest predisposing cause to damage is the use of forceps. When a recognised third degree tear occurs, 85 percent of women have persistent structural sphincter defects and one half are still symptomatic, despite a primary repair at the time of delivery [4]. Structural damage associated with childbirth is more important than neurological factors, the latter appearing to coincide with structural damage rather than being the cause of incontinence [5].

The damage which occurs during childbirth affects the anterior anal sphincter. Most commonly the external anal sphincter is disrupted. This is believed to be due to an unrecognised extension of a tear. If the tear is more extensive, it may also involve the internal anal sphincter. Occasionally the internal anal sphincter alone appears to be disrupted, and this may relate to a shearing force on this thin muscle, rather than a direct tear.

The second commonest cause of incontinence leading to referral to a diagnostic unit is faecal incontinence following anal surgery. The anal sphincter may have been damaged unavoidably, such as during anal fistula surgery, or avoidably as a result of anal sphincterotomy for anal fissure or anal dilatation.

Other causes of trauma include motor bike accidents, war injuries, and unwanted sexual penetration. Motor bike and war injuries can result in major anatomical sphincter disruption, which varies from patient to patient. Unwanted sexual penetration can lead to internal sphincter disruption, and occasionally to associated external sphincter disruption. Most commonly the internal anal sphincter is fragmented and thinned [1, 2]. Occasionally, however, trauma leads to an intact but grossly hypertrophied and weak internal sphincter.

Neuropathic damage

Neuropathic sphincter damage is probably much less common than was previously believed. Most patients with incontinence and evidence of neurological damage in the pelvic floor have associated structural damage, with the latter accounting for the functional abnormality.

Degenerative, congenital, myopathic and neurological disorders

A number of primary disorders which involve degeneration of intestinal smooth muscle are also associated with degeneration of the smooth muscle internal anal sphincter. This is seen in some patients with gastrointestinal involvement with primary systemic sclerosis (scleroderma) and some patients with chronic idiopathic intestinal pseudoobstruction due to visceral myopathy

Faecal incontinence is also seen in some neurological disorders, and can be a common and major cause of disability. It occurs in approximately 30 % of patients with multiple sclerosis, and a high proportion of patients with spinal injury.

Patients who have corrective surgery as a neonate or infant for congenital imperforate anus, or Hirschsprung's disease, can experience faecal incontinence in later childhood or adolescence. This can be due to associated rectal abnormalities, deficient sphincter muscle, or failure to position the bowel through the sphincter ring at surgery in the neonatal period, so that it is not surrounded by striated external anal sphincter muscle.

Characterising the sphincter abnormality

Accurate characterisation of bowel and sphincter function is essential to select patients who are likely to benefit from surgery, to define the type of surgery required, and to give some guide to prognosis. It is important to elucidate the extent, frequency and nature of incontinence.

Investigations provide information about sphincter.

(1) **Function**. Manometry is helpful in defining the strength of each of the sphincter muscles. Measurements of sensory function provide some indication about possible neurological disease.

(2) **Structure**. Anal endosonography, and to a lesser extent MRI, have revolutionised the ability to characterise sphincter anatomy, disruptions and degeneration.

Decision making is then based on the constellation of history, functional and anatomical studies. Each of these is well validated and proven to influence management and outcome.

Surgery for « neuropathic » injury

The traditional operation for incontinence which was believed to be due to nerve damage and weakness due to progressive denervation has been the post anal repair. This operation involved plicating the sphincter muscles posteriorly, lengthening the anal canal and increasing the anorectal angle.

Although this operation helped patients in the short term, the long term results have been more disappointing. In a study which examined the outcome 5 to 8 years after surgery, only a quarter of patients were continent for solids and liquids [6].

With the advent of anal endosonography, and the recognition that many of these patients have structural damage, there is no longer a clear role for this operation.

Surgery for sphincter trauma

Obstetric sphincter damage

Sphincter repair for incontinence following childbirth is a worthwhile operation, leading to a high success rate and a major improvement in many patients symptoms.

The anterior damage can involve one or both of the sphincter muscles. Characterisation is dependent on ultrasound. The operation involves making an adequate incision to expose the ends of the ruptured striated muscle, then overlapping the two ends of the muscle along the length of the anal canal. If the internal anal sphincter is also disrupted, an attempt should be made to pick up the ends of this muscle in the repair ; the internal sphincter is too thin and delicate to repair separately.

In the largest published study to date, 55 patients with obstetric related faecal incontinence underwent repair; 32 had incontinence after delivery and 23 had late onset incontinence. Anal endosonography and physiological tests were performed before and after surgery. After a median of 15 months (range 6-36), 42 patients were improved, 11 were not improved, and 2 were awaiting colostomy closure. Improved patients had a greater increase in postoperative squeeze pressure (20 vs 5 cm H_2O, $p = 0.05$) and endosonographically the external sphincter (EAS) was more frequently intact (intact EAS ring 32/35 vs 5/11, $p = 0.003$). Patients with an intact EAS had higher postoperative squeeze pressures (intact vs not intact EAS : 50 vs 20 cm H_2O, $p = 0.004$). The late onset group were older than those who presented soon after childbirth (median 59 vs 32 years, $p < 0.001$), had longer pudendal nerve terminal motor latencies (2.3 vs 2.1 ms, $p = 0.027$), but other measurements and continence grade did not differ. Repair failure was related to persistent EAS defects. Late onset incontinence, even with a prolonged pudendal nerve terminal motor latency, did not preclude a good outcome. A colostomy is not necessary to cover the repair.

Non-obstetric non-surgical perineal trauma

Patients who have experienced perineal, and in particular anal, trauma, due to war injuries or motor bike accidents, can often do well if the injury is well characterised. In one study, over a twelve year period 65 patients were assessed for post traumatic assessment of the anal sphincters and continence mechanism. All patients were continent before their trauma. Using clinical examination, manometry, concentric needle EMG and most recently anal endosonography, external sphincter defects were present in 56 patients and absent in 9. Of the former group of patients, 52 underwent overlapping sphincter repair. At a median follow-up of 12 months, a good result (continence grade 1+2) was achieved in 36 patients (69 %), a poor result (continence grade 3+4) occurred in 10 patients (19 %), and 6 patients were lost to follow up. A good result was associated with a significant increase ($p = 0.017$) in resting pressure (median increase 15 cm H_2O) and with a significant increase ($p = 0.001$) in squeeze pressure (median increase 35 cm H_2O). In the postoperative assessment, three patients with a poor outcome were shown to have a second unsuspected contralateral sphincter defect which had not been repaired. In conclusion, physiological and endosonographic investigation combined with late surgical repair leads to a good outcome in the majority of patients with traumatic sphincter damage.

Isolated internal anal sphincter disruption

Isolated internal anal sphincter disruption is not amenable to simple surgical repair. The muscle is too thin and the repair is not maintained.

Surgery for internal sphincter damage or degeneration extensive sphincter injury, or as part of restorative surgery

In certain circumstances the sphincter muscles are not amenable to simple surgical repair. This is always the case in isolated degenerative or structural abnormalities involving the internal anal sphincter alone. It is also the case when there is extensive disruption of the external anal sphincter. Other situations include sphincter excision as part of an abdominoperineal excision for cancer, or extensive previous surgery for conditions such as complex fistulae or sepsis, and complex congenital abnormalities.

Under such circumstances it is necessary to create an artificial sphincter high pressure zone. This can be performed using striated muscle transposed to replace the normal sphincter muscles. Muscles which have been used to do this include gluteus maximus and gracilis. The operation can be performed unilaterally or bilaterally.

Striated muscle contains a mixture of type 1 and type 2 fibres, responsible for sustained and fast twitch contraction. The external anal sphincter is unusual in containing a high proportion of sustained activity muscle fibres. However the transplanted muscles do not contain such a ratio of type 1 to type 2 fibres and therefore fatigue quickly. To overcome this problem these muscles have been artificially electrically stimulated long term. In addition to maintaining contraction in the muscle, this stimulation also causes a transformation of many of the muscle fibres to a slow twitch fatigue-resistant type (type 1) [7].

The gracilis transplant with stimulation, otherwise known as the dynamic graciloplasty, has been used for the treatment of idiopathic incontinence, for patients with congenital anorectal malformation, and for patients after cancer abdomino-perineal resection. In the largest and best study published to date, 52 patients were prospectively evaluated with interview, manometry, and quality of life assessment [8]. Seventy three percent were continent after a median follow-up of 2 years. The median bowel frequency decreased from five to two per day, and the median time defaecation could be postponed increased from 9 seconds to 19 minutes. Patients with a successful outcome became less anxious than those in whom it failed, and significantly improved their effectiveness in performing tasks around the home, personal relationships, sexual function, and social life. They also became significantly less isolated socially.

The artificial sphincter offers exciting prospects for patients with incontinence in whom sphincter repair is not possible. Only a small number of patients have been treated in the published studies to date, using a device designed for the urethral sphincter. The device consists of an inflatable cuff that is placed around the anal canal, an implanted reservoir, and a valve-pump which is placed in the scrotum or labia. Using the subcutaneous valve allows the cuff to be deflated for defaecation. A range of devices designed for the anal sphincter are currently undergoing evaluation.

Some patients have incontinence due to sphincter weakness but circumferentially intact sphincter muscle rings. It may be possible to activate these muscles by providing chronic stimulation *via* the normal nerve supply. A preliminary report of three patients has suggested that electrostimulation to the spinal nerve roots may improve striated muscle function. Two patients regained full continence, while one had substantial improvement [9].

Stoma

For some patients drug therapy has failed and extensive anal surgery has either failed, is not appropriate, or is not technically feasible. A stoma should be considered. It is a relatively simple operation which provides a dramatic improvement of quality of life for some patients.

References

1. Engel AF, Kamm MA, Bartram CI. Unwanted anal penetration as a physical cause for faecal incontinence. *Eur J Gastroenterol Hepatol* 1995; 7: 65-7.
2. Sultan AH, Kamm MA, Hudson CN, Bartram CI. Anal sphincter disruption during vaginal delivery. *N Engl J Med* 1993; 329: 1905-11.
3. Sultan AH, Kamm MA, Bartram CI, Hudson CN. Third degree obstetric anal sphincter tears. Risk factors and outcome of primary repair. *Br Med J* 1994; 308: 887-91.

4. Kamm MA. Obstetric damage and faecal incontinenc. *Lancet* 1994; 344: 730-3.
5. Angel AF, Kamm MA, Bartram CI, Nicholls RJ. Relationship of symptoms in faecal incontinence to specific sphincter abnormalities. *Int J Colorect Dis* 1995; 10: 152-5.
6. Setti Carraro P, Kamm MA, Nicholls RJ. Long term results of postanal repair for neurogenic faecal incontinence. *Br J Surg* 1994; 81: 140-4.
7. George BD, Williams NS, Patel J, Swash M, Watkins ES. Physiological and histochemical adaptation of the electrically stimulated gracilis muscle to neoanal sphincter function. *Br J Surg* 1993; 80: 1342-6.
8. Baeten CGMI, Geerdes BP, Adang EMM, Heineman E, Konsten J, Engel GL, Ketser ADM, Spaans F, Soeters PB. Anal dynamic graciloplasty in the treatment of intractable fecal incontinence. *N Engl J Med* 1995; 332: 1600-5.
9. Matzel KE, Stadelmaier U, Hohenfellner M, Gall FP. Electrical stimulation of scacral spinal nerves for treatment of faecal incontinence. *Lancet* 1995; 346: 1124-7.

Achevé d'imprimer par Corlet, Imprimeur, S.A.
14110 Condé-sur-Noireau (France)
N° d'Imprimeur : 19684 - Dépôt légal : octobre 1996

Imprimé en C.E.E.